OVERCOMING

FEAR

Challenging Our Greatest Disability

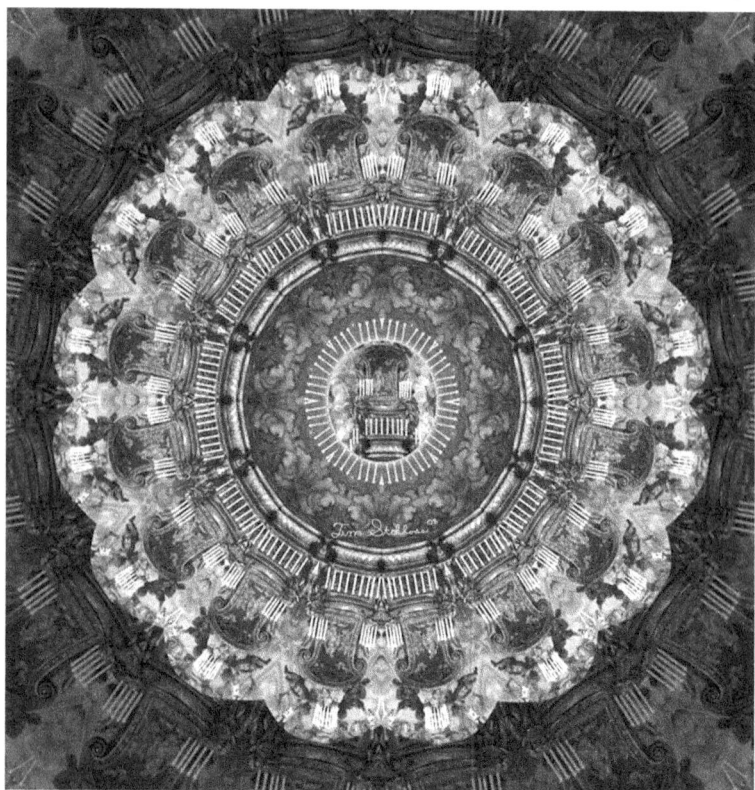

Mandala. Tim Stoklosa, 2008

OVERCOMING

FEAR

Challenging Our Greatest Disability

COSTA NDAYISABYE *and*
TIMOTHY STOKLOSA

Great Life Press
Rye, New Hampshire
2015

Softcover ISBN: 978-1-938394-15-7
Ebook ISBN: 978-1-938394-16-4
Library of Congress Control Number: 2015940068
published by
Great Life Press, Rye, New Hampshire
www.greatlifepress.com

Front cover art by Timothy Stoklosa
Back cover photo by Grace Peirce

Interviews and conversations recorded in this book are used with the permission and consent of the interviewees.

Contents

Acknowledgments

I am highly grateful to God who inspired me to write this second book and gave me courage and strength to successfully achieve it.

I am grateful to my wife Bernadette Ndayisabye, my kids Yves-Claude, Gentle, Queen and Denise who supported me with prayers and relaxed time to put my ideas on paper.

Thank you to my mother Marthe, who encouraged me to focus on my task as she was recovering from her short stroke.

I am thankful to Grace Peirce, the owner of Great Life Press, who helped refine this work to a clearer writing standard, helped us to discover the right title, and created the cover design featuring Tim Stoklosa's art.

This book would not be a mind-changing one without the contribution of my co-author Timothy Stoklosa and his mother Karen Anderson, who show the world that FEAR is manageable; consequently we have the ability to overcome FEAR.

I am also thankful to the following friends and leaders who provided valuable insights to me along the way: Alexandre Mejat, PhD in Biology, the Muscular Dystrophy Association of France; the Muscular Dystrophy Association of Westbrook, Maine; Dwight Wendell, English and Philosophy teacher in Central Okanagan school district of British Columbia, Canada; Pei-Ming Sun of Indiana, who gave her time and her heart to contribute to this book; Artiste Dennis C. Johnson who spent hours straightening the language of this book; Brenda Lowe and The One Person Project, who through love committed to give her time and heart to a vulnerable community in Africa; Janviere Uwumikiza, though lying down on your bed always, your mind travels and your love reaches so many hearts; Pastor Jeff and Darilynn Tarbox, founders of New Life Church Biddeford, Maine, you are always in our hearts with your straightforward teachings of the word of God; Janine Giles from Canmore in Alberta, Canada, who I hold in my heart for her wisdom; Carrie Haldy and the entire Hilderman family of Saskatchewan, Canada; family friends Nancy and Jim Colby of Kennebunk, Maine, whose love toward my family shows the power of Oneness; Rob, Carol, and Stephanie Marocco, always be blessed for your love; our lovely family friends in Texas, Charles and Teresa Kennedy, Dean and Cissy Sitton, our inspirational peoples, Tommy Politz, Brad Clark, Mark Zimmerman and the entire Hillside Christian Church, for their non-discriminating welcome to all the community; and our love goes to Pastor Ronnie Nemoede and all of our lovely friends from the Village Park Church; and ALL who supported the funding of this project.

Also my gratitude goes to all the inspirational people and businesses, including Naren and Sono King of Crystal Castle in Australia, www.crystalcastle.com.au, who provide tremendous love and support; my friend Byron Katie, the founder of The Work, who inspired me to write my first book; all the friends of The Work; Bartlomiej and Heather Skorupa and the entire team from Groundwork Opportunity, San Francisco, California, for your love toward vulnerable communities around the globe.

I thank all my friends, including those who may not be not mentioned here—I hold you all in my heart always.

— Costa Ndayisabye

To start I would like to thank God and Jesus Christ for all the blessings, mercy, and salvation they provide. "And we know that God causes all things to work together for good to those who love God, to those who are called according to His purpose."

I want to thank Costa Ndayisabye for his friendship, love, and support. I am very honored to have had the privilege of working with him to write this book. I would also like to acknowledge and thank all the family and friends who have loved and supported me over the years. Most of all my mom Karen Anderson, grandmother Clare Anderson, my father Tim Stoklosa, stepmother Marybeth Stoklosa, and stepfather Roy Cohn. My caregivers and friends: Connie Johnson, Jane Garza, Dawn Munson, Charity Meserve, Tiffany Crockett, Devin DeLaite, Sharon Price, and Bonney Grover. And my friends Scott Davies, Tom Shaw, Tom Bennet, Trisha Summers Edwards, Mark Mueller, and Simon Garza.

— Timothy Stoklosa

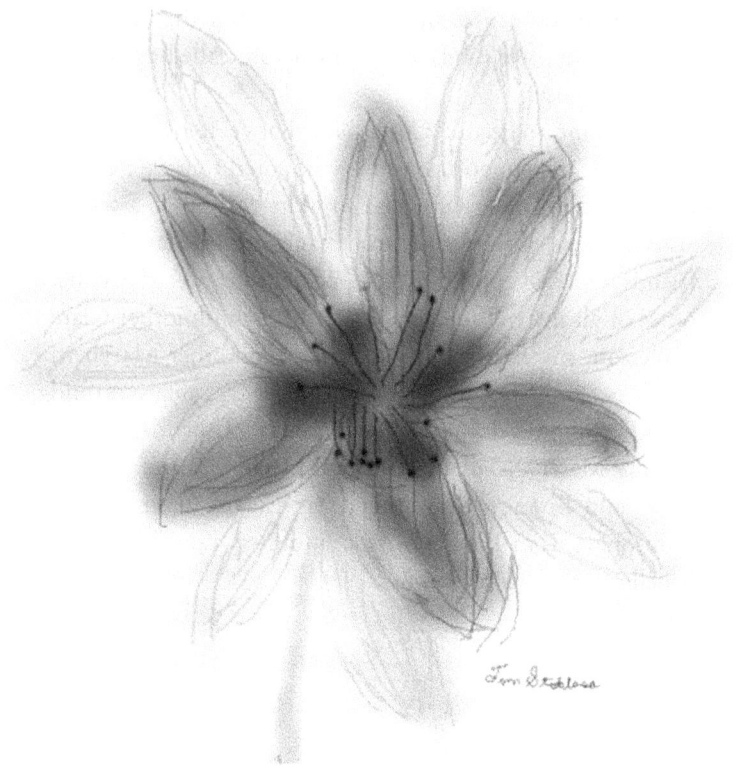

Preface

Everyone is capable of an enlightened view of his or her or another's interpretation of physical attributes. It is a matter of becoming aware that our minds are projecting to the outside something different from what is really there. I believe this book, with a Foreword by the mother of a young man with Duchenne muscular dystrophy, may empower the reader's understanding of what it is like to discover the ability within us, by living the Present, without being disturbed by negative thoughts and feelings that interfere with the love and peace we deserve. What we see is not the complete picture of who we are.

"Are you from Thrive School?" a former governor of the State of Maine asked, upon meeting this beautiful guy in a wheelchair named Tim Stoklosa. Thrive School in Maine is an educational support program for mentally challenged youth with emotional and behavioral difficulties.

"I didn't care. That was the way he thought I was," Tim said. "It is sometimes bad to picture, or judge someone by a stereotypical perception," Tim added. "Being wheelchair-bound does not at all mean someone has mental challenges." Yet many people automatically jump to this conclusion. People often make wrong assumptions about the appearance of persons with severe disability in wheelchairs. Even prominent people from government and other places of "power" can make this same mistake.

Maybe I, Costa, or you, or him, or her—have made the same confused observation.

Everyone has his or her own life experience; this

story about Tim can take you on a journey deep inside yourself to realize how wonderful you are, how you can be, by living the Present without being affected by our stressful past. Our past "story" happens in a glimpse of time and its present impact will depend on how our mind gives meaning to that story. Let us also be more mindful when complaining, simply because we may be mistakenly doing so.

When people used to ask me about events in my past, I would resentfully relate the situations I had experienced. Reliving old stories is a big part of life for many people. We dwell so much on negative experiences that happened to us in the past that we end up losing hope and living hopelessly. We should be careful that we are not too attached to our old stories. Sometimes we agree to let our minds be ruled by our old stories. We agree to dwell on our grief-stricken past moments and forget the power and positive possibilities of today.

When I share with people my approach to living in the Present, while at the same time not forgetting, but carefully using the past, I enjoy seeing how people discover that their ability to do something for themselves is Present right NOW within them. It's a matter of noticing that what is outside of us is simply something our minds may project onto, and its only value is what we give it. We unquestionably can do something special and valuable for our own lives by recognizing that the power of peace God has placed within us gives us the ability to maximize the possibilities of our being.

While you are holding this book in your hands, take a moment to realize the power that is dwelling within you and take a deep journey inside yourself for its wonderful consciousness. This is the internal power that opens our connection to true peace. It is the power that helps to focus our being and on our "I" instead of thinking that our body or something outside of us holds the peace we need in order to enjoy the Present. It is the power that helps to stop all the blames we place on our relatives, our friends, and the universe—the power to put a spotlight on our strengths, which can help us change our lives into lovely ones.

—Costa Ndayisabye

Foreword

The first time I held Timothy Charles (Timmy) in the autumn of 1983; I gazed at his perfectly round pumpkin face and felt the deepest joy of my life. I had never felt such a profound happiness. He was warm and rosy with tiny transparent fingernails which I carefully untangled from his felt swaddling, artfully formed utensils which seemed miraculous in their tiny creation. I remember inspecting him from tip to toe, whispering, "Hello baby boy, I've been waiting to meet you, and here you are, so perfect and real." I counted fingers, toenails, and ears, two sturdy legs and one belly button, taking an exhaustive inventory. Nothing could be missing. I inhaled him, holding him as if he were made of the most precious material in the world. His innocence and dependence were absolute and complete.

On that day heartbreak entered my world, but it felt like joy. If only I'd known the ambush to come. The day was November the 8th, 1983. Little did I know that in this perfect moment of sunlight and joy, lurking in my DNA was the secret to his physical undoing. I felt the deepest sense of trickery and betrayal—that my baby could appear so healthy and strong, when tucked deep within his double helix was the secret to his muscles unraveling.

Diagnosed with Duchenne muscular dystrophy at age three, he has grown from baby Timothy, to little Timmy, to a young man named Tim. He is no longer swaddled in a baby bunting but his dependence is nonetheless complete.

On December 8th 2004, Tim is twenty-one years and one month old. His massive power wheelchair holds his fleshy body in place and allows him his own freedom in place of sturdy legs. His hands are claw-like with little utility. His round face, bright green eyes, smooth skin and full lips are trusting and open. A bodhisattva. A calm presence. He touches you. But now he is leaving behind all he has ever known. No longer glowing orange to yellow, my world hardened to gun-gray metal.

Today we take an inventory of Tim's belongings. In a giant black duffle we have packed his flannel sweat pants, XXL shirts, sweaters, Hoyer pad, tube socks, video games and DVDs. He is leaving home for the first time in his life, the same home where he has lived since birth. The house where three times a night I rise and turn his body and stretch his legs, lift his arms and do all the mid-night motions for him that he cannot do for himself. 11:00 p.m., 2:00 a.m., 5:00 a.m. I have not slept through the night for twenty-one years.

I pace outside the nursing home; my heart beating 130 beats per minute. I circle the concrete parking lot unable to follow Tim and his care attendant into the lobby. I stand by our midnight blue Ride-away van under a steel gray sky and wonder how I can leave him behind. How can I drive away and leave him in this place. I stare up at a barracks with five even floors, a massive red brick rectangle with small vinyl windows. The nursing home. It could be a prison if it were surrounded in barbed wire.

My mother had died three months earlier. I lost my job. The funding was cut to provide homecare.

The discharge nurse says, "I'm sorry but he is no longer a child. Our services terminate when he turns twenty-one years of age. He's an adult now. You'll need to find other arrangements."

My boyfriend leaves. Tim's father moves away. Without help the gunmetal weight takes us to the bottom.

"Yes, there is the nursing home. There are other young men living there." The care coordinator makes it sound like a bargain.

Barely breathing, my skin feels thin and I feel as if I am floating unhinged in the ether. If you asked me what color—I'd have to say, "No color. Just air." I am suspended above the parking lot for as long as I can go without air,— then I fall, slam—back to earth.

Jane comes running, "Karen, come on. Intake is waiting for you. You have to sign the papers."

I walk in tentatively and see Tim aglow, waiting for me. He is excited. His friends have all gone off to college and now it is his turn for freedom. He takes care of me.

"It's okay mom. It's time for me to be on my own."

He's excited. It's an adventure. But really he's just hoping to meet some young pretty nurse. I warm when I see his spark which is really a twinkling inner light, but then I'm assaulted by the smells—a mixture of antiseptics, cleaning solutions, urine, and aging bodies. I am struck by a new realization. This is where people go to die. I look left and right and see wrinkled bodies slumped in wheelchairs parked sideways to the sun. There are no young folk to be found. I choke back tears and sign the papers. Then we go upstairs. Tim loads into the elevator with the in-take nurse and Jane. I take the stairs. I can't imagine riding in a gun-metal vault to the second floor.

In the lobby of 2-South I am again assaulted by the stinging odors of bodily fluids, sour food and bleach. Large Naugahyde recliners hold comatose bodies that could be corpses. There is a fake Christmas tree in the corner with plastic baubles and colored lights. We follow the in-take nurse down the bland green hall to Tim's room. We pass by whitewashed rooms with bodies strapped to wheelchairs or lying under coarse sheets in their beds. Rounding a bend we hear loud incoherent moans coming from a heavy bald woman in her bed, clutching a baby-doll. "Oh that's Peggy. Hi Peggy." The nurse chimes.

Tim's new quarters holds two identical hospital beds, two small bureaus, two night stands and one very large TV. Lyland, a young man of thirty, paralyzed from the neck down, had been a member of a prominent motor-cycle gang prior to smashing into a brick wall at high speed (so the nurse whispers to us). The volume is turned up high and hard-eyed Lyland, with dirty-blond hair lies in bed watching cars zoom around a track. The sound is deafening but he cannot lower the volume without help. The nurse introduces Tim to Lyland and they acknowledge one another with sideways glances. We pull the suspended flowered curtain between the beds and look around. The smell is relentlessly acrid. It is very hot

"We keep the heat very high. Without movement many of our patients get cold." The nurse speaks in a little whisper voice.

I take off my sweater and lay it on the windowsill and stare down into the parking lot. I want to run away to make my heart stop pounding. Hot tears well up and a hard clay mound forms at the back of my throat. I fake smiles at everyone. I study my only son. Tim is at peace. I can see it in his sparkling green eyes. He is strong and free at last in a mere one hundred square feet of pungent living space.

Tim is ready to find his place in this new world. He

seems unfazed by the whisper of death in every corner, where nurses sleep-walk the aisles, pacing in and out of rooms. I look at Tim and study his composure. He is as open and trusting as a small child. I remember one social worker describing young men with DMD as absolutely normal with extraordinary physical challenges. Tim wants to grow up. Tim wants his independence. At a time when his peer group has left home to make their way in the world Tim has become even more dependent. He cannot walk, lift his arms, dress himself, bathe himself, feed himself or do any tiny task we all take for granted. His call to grow is in direct contradiction to his physical decline and this nursing home is his hope for self-actualization.

Tim lived at the nursing home from December 2004 to May 2005. Sadly, in the state of Maine, once you turn twenty-one, you lose homecare services funded under the Maternal Child Health program. Tim was ineligible to live in a community group home because his IQ was too high. To live in a group home you must have a developmental disability, which is measured as an IQ below 70.

On his final day at the nursing home he was taken by ambulance to Maine Medical Center where he spent two months in intensive care. He'd lost over thirty pounds and was close to death. He had been sent to that nursing home to die.

Since 2005 a loving team of nurses and aides have nursed Tim back to health. He now lives in his own apartment decorated with fall pumpkins, with his cat Zoey and around-the-clock care. His new freedom came at the cost of becoming ventilator dependent. Thankfully there is not a nursing home in the state of Maine that provides ventilator care. He has gained back more than thirty pounds, is close to finishing a Bachelor of Arts Degree in Graphic Design from the University of Maine and continues to sparkle and break hearts. I no longer feel that deep sense of trickery, which came with his diagnosis. I have grown inwardly rich and glow from gunmetal gray to violet to blue to green, red and blaze orange yellow in the presence of my son and his unraveling double helix.

    —Karen Anderson

Introduction

The life of the gentleman who is going to be our bona fide mirror of focus, who cultivates peace despite physical weakness and without any complaint, is that of one Timothy Stoklosa, otherwise known as Tim, which is what we shall call him throughout the rest of this book. During summertime afternoons, if you happen to be around Ocean Park, close to the Pines retirement community on Manor Street in the town of Old Orchard Beach, Maine, or maybe in downtown Old Orchard Beach, you may meet a man in a wheelchair who appears immediately to be unique due to the physical appearance of his person. Bound to an electric wheelchair, with a constant ventilator attached on the back, and a long tube ending with a pipe close to his mouth that supplies extra oxygen—these are the tools that support this wonderful man in his mobility. Someone always accompanies him and he gives a nice smile to those he meets—especially friends and relatives and anyone who will say "hi" to him.

My journey with Tim, who has Duchenne muscular dystrophy, started with continuously challenging observations. The time I spent with him helped me to understand that physical disability does not necessarily mean mind disability.

I find some similarities between Tim's perspective of thinking and mine, in regards to the real peace that opens the door to the reality of our being.

Better life is all about peace, the real peace that comes from deep inside of us. What our body struggles with, starts with the projections of our mind. When our consciousness is consumed by fear we do not care for ourselves, and cannot value others.

Tim's mom, Karen Anderson, is a very important person in his life. She is a mother with passion to provide love and also a picture of humankind that we all need. In my early experience with him, I noticed that whenever he had anything to share, whether it was a concern or happy event, he would ask, "Can I call my mom?"

When you meet them, you will see how one's presence is very important to the other's life. There is a lovely connection all the time.

This is the ultimate role that a mother plays in the life of someone she loves. A proverb in my language, Kinyarwanda, states: "The only person you can lose and you will not find again is your mother." She cannot be replaced.

A big fear that can be experienced is fear of getting into conflict with one's mother. A friend asked me one day "Costa, what would happen to you if your mother does harm to you?" I responded that I would focus on what led her to do that to me and then consider myself as my mom's caregiver.

If we need to learn about relevant stress management, including perseverance and forgiveness, we should observe the life connection between mother and child.

Karen Anderson is the closest person to Tim and has dedicated her life to her lovely son. She has a Bachelor of Science in accounting, and a Bachelor of Arts in philosophy, with a minor in creative writing, from the University of Southern Maine. While compiling this book, Karen was a Controller for MARC (Marlen Abela Restaurant Corporation) and she traveled a lot for her job.

I wanted to know much more about the wonderful man Timothy and how he lives a life in its fullness today despite the physical difficulties he has, so I spoke with his mom.

Costa: When did it first happen for Tim to be in a wheelchair?

Karen: Timmy [as Karen likes calling her son] was diagnosed at age two and a half with a genetic defect that causes Duchenne muscular dystrophy. The genetic coding of his muscles is missing the recipe for the formation of dystrophin. This lack first causes muscle weakness and then total failure of all muscle systems, including the lungs. He was born with the ability to walk, and did so until he was nine years old. He began falling down a lot from the time he was seven, until he went into a wheelchair.

Costa: What was your reaction when you first realized what was happening?

Karen: When I first found out that Tim had muscular dystrophy I was devastated and literally cried for months. I cried for days on end and could not stop mourning the sadness of his fate. I prayed all the time and asked God for the strength to understand this cruel disease. After time, and many, many hours of prayer, I eventually felt very touched by God and understood in a profound way that Tim's disease was not a mistake and that it was part of a plan that God had for all of us, and that we would all grow and change for the better as a result of this awesome fate.

Costa: What impression did you get when you saw Tim for the first time in a wheelchair?

Karen: Actually, it was a rather joyful day when Tim first used a wheelchair. His third grade classmates were part of the process of getting Tim ready to use a wheelchair. All the children met in small groups before Tim's chair was delivered so that they could share their feelings and not be frightened of his new dependence on a wheelchair. They were so excited when the day arrived that Tim showed up in his new chair and they clapped and took turns pushing him around his school. His classmates were so loving and excited for Tim that it was really a fun time. Also, he had been falling a lot so it was a relief that he would not hurt himself any longer.

Costa: Tell our readers the two most sorrowful stories you encountered while taking care of Tim.

Karen: The first was when Tim spent a couple of weeks in a children's hospital when he was undergoing tests for his diagnosis when he was almost three years old. He was in the neurology wing of the hospital and shared a room with a five-year-old with a brain tumor. In fact, most of the children on the floor had brain tumors and many would die very young. It was a sad and overwhelming place and I had such a hard time getting used to the fact that Tim was not healthy and would not be a normal child.

The next most sorrowful time was when Tim went to live in the nursing home at age twenty-one.

Costa: What are some of the wonderful souvenirs you have kept from your son Tim's childhood?

Karen: We have saved all of Tim's artwork from his youth. He was able to draw by hand then, and we have saved all of his hand-drawn art. We have photos from when he could walk and run. There are several pictures of Tim in the newspapers. He was a very photogenic young boy.

Costa: Did you have any sense of hope for Tim's life when he was so young?

Karen: I prayed and prayed to God to understand Tim's affliction. And God answered our prayers. Tim's illness is not a mistake. It is part of God's plan. Everyone who touches Tim's life is moved and altered by his grace and strength. He can get very depressed and angry at what has been taken from him. All he wants is to love and be loved. I don't understand how he has the strength to live his life. I am in complete awe of his strength. I see him as a savior who is sacrificed so others can be lifted up in his presence. He breaks my heart every day. And he keeps me very, very close to God for the courage to understand his illness. But yes, it is very painful to witness his struggles.

Costa: As a mom, what was your strategy to raise Tim from his early years up to now?

Karen: Tim has been loved and yes, spoiled!! They say spoiling is when you do something for a child that they can do for themselves. And often I probably did too much for him! At one point he wanted to kill himself, he was so sad and frustrated. I took him to the priest at our church. They spent a lot of time together, and Tim found the courage to face his trials. I often dragged him to God kicking and screaming when he was a child. He didn't want to go. He was angry and didn't believe in God. But we kept showing up and kept praying and begging God for help. I tell Tim all the time we are both physical and spiritual beings. Your spirit is stronger than your body and you can transcend the body with your spirit. His spirit frees him when he creates his art. His art is pure spirit. I have always encouraged him to make art. I took him out of his high school in Old Orchard and sent him to Thornton Academy because of their amazing art program. So yes—art set Tim FREE!! Art and spirit and GOD!

Costa: Do you think Tim contributed to the life that he's living now?

Karen: Yes—Tim's artwork is his life and his calling. His art is so pure and beautiful, and makes so many people happy.

Costa: From your observation as his mom, who do you think he is today?

Karen: He is a young man who struggles every day to find love. My greatest prayer for my son is that he finds a woman to love who will love him back.

Costa: Does Tim inspire you and your life today?

Karen: Of course. He is pure heartbreak and pure inspiration. He keeps me close to God and spirit.

Costa: Are you satisfied with the way people in the community treat your son or other people with muscular dystrophy?

Karen: Yes. You really get to understand a person by their reaction to Tim and how they either reject or embrace his life. There have been some cruel young women who have not been kind to him. But on the other hand there are people who are so loving and generous. One who comes to mind is COSTA!!

Costa: What kind of image would you wish individuals to consider when meeting people with muscular dystrophy?

Karen: People with muscular dystrophy are perfectly normal people with overwhelming physical challenges! They just want to be heard and embraced as a vital part of their community.

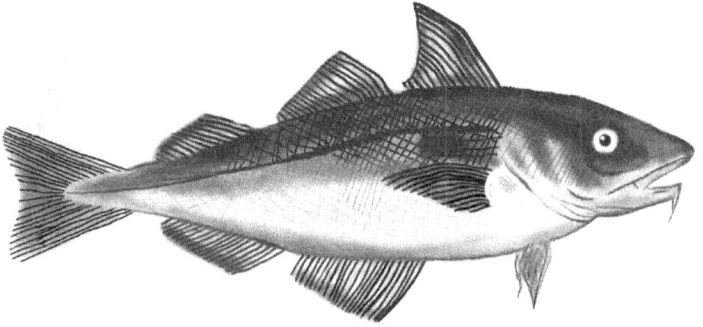

Jim Stidham

Inquiring Minds Ask: That Thought, Does it Bring Peace, or Hatred?

As I wrote in my first book, *The Work That Brings Peace in Me*, I was the type of person who was much connected to "the grief-stricken moments that happened to me and my family." I was always comparing my fearful past to my present life without seeing the ability—the power—that dwelled within me.

I went through an inquiry process with myself and questioned my mind: "Whose business is it when I am attached to my stressful stories?" Then I discovered that the true life is THE PRESENT ONE and the past one is simply Story.

I have never encouraged my mind to forget the past story, but before becoming engrossed in it, I take time to balance and consider what it is going to bring to me: Peace or anger? Peace or stress? That balancing process is called The Work/Inquiry. After the inquiry process, I can continue to indulge my story or I can choose to ignore it and its influence before making any important decision. Note that when our minds are fearful, we tightly bind ourselves to stressful stories that happened to us in the past. Any experience that happened in the past, even in the past minute, is Story. That is what I have learned time after time. Be careful and critical while using Story.

The more carefully our Story is used, the more peacefully we can live.

Some of the stories that we are attached to can ruin our lives while others can give strength, depending on the way we perceive them.

I met a friend in Canada who was very attached to the death of her husband. When the memory of her husband's death came, she fell into crisis and couldn't do anything. She was surrounded by the image of seeing her husband leaving her. One day we shared a long phone call. The subject of our conversation was the celebration of the anniversary of her husband's death. She was afraid and anxious about how it would be for her during that day of anniversary! I reminded her that she still holds a lot of wonderful moments that she had with her husband before he died. I added that with a simple shift within her, she could find a positive way to celebrate. She decided to cook for the guests the foods her husband liked the most, serve the drink her husband liked drinking, and share with the guests some jokes or relevant experiences she had enjoyed with her always loving, but now deceased husband.

Our mind's weakness due to what has happened to us shouldn't stop us from using the internal force that dwells within us.

It's when our minds become fearful that we aren't paying attention and lose control of our focus, and live hopelessly.

A fearful mind likes projecting blame for its confusions on something outside of itself and pretends to obtain internal peace from that. Examples of these confusions can include:

- "I am miserable because my mom doesn't care about me at all." (One of my solutions is to

believe that keeping my distance from my mom will give me peace.)
- "Since I married her/him, I have never been peaceful. She/he doesn't really love me."
- "My body is weak; it can't do anything."

An educated person will try to calm his or her stress or anguish using books, articles, and other academic notions, projecting the answer to the outside! Is that where the peace you want really dwells?

- "He or she made me miserable or frustrated."
  (Does he or she really control my peace?)

The question to ask is: "Whose business is it when I am confused?"

The short answer is: Mine.

I am the one. This is the point of discovery of my own power over my life in the Present.

With the power of the Present, we can all value who we are and what we have today.

Adventures with Tim

The inspiring story of Karen and her son Tim, who was growing up with steadily degrading physical abilities, was witnessed by a lot of people who had known Tim since he was a little boy. They saw all of the physical changes that were totally opposite to his mind, which is full of both strength and aptitudes. I approached Holly, Tim's long-time neighbor and friend, and asked her to describe him.

Prior to describing him, Holly wrote down "Timmy":

Art saves
Montessori concept of function
Purpose
Community ties
Advocacy - mom
Technology
Vision
Connection to something larger
Courage
Determination
Live life
Fulfillment on his terms

Holly: I've known Timmy for as long as I can remember. I recall his attempts at a tricycle, pedaling up Mass. Ave. in Old Orchard Beach here in Maine, with Grandma Claire close at hand. An extended family unit played a deep role in his life. Tim's grandmother was an ever-present entity in his life and she was the one who filled in the gaps for his mom. Many felt her loss.

I watched Tim walk independently, then walk with the aid of a walker. From there, the disease progressed and he transitioned to a manual wheelchair and then finally, an electric one. I've witnessed his feet no longer able to wear shoes, until his Achilles tendons were cut. I witnessed the arrival of his puff ventilator, giving him the oxygen he needed, on his own terms, thus protecting what independent lung function he still possesses. And then last summer's valiant effort to eradicate the C-Diff [*Clostridium difficile*] in his system, by means of fecal transplant [fecal microbiota transplantation (FMT) is the best treatment for C-Diff bacterial disease].

I watched Tim's skill with his art progress, yet reduce in size as the movement of his hand lessened with the progression of the disease. I remember one piece; a drawing in pencil, made from a series of two-inch squares and then pieced together to make the whole. At the time of this drawing, a one-inch radius was all the movement he had in his hand. Now he depends entirely on the use of a computer and its mouse.

Thinking of Tim, the phrase "Art Saves," comes to life for me. Art gives him purpose, fulfillment, and a means of full expression. Art connects him to something larger, a community, and something beyond.

As for Karen, all children should know such devotion. She supports Tim in his quest for independence, but she remains close at hand. Her ability to uncover new treatment options for him, I believe, has extended his life and has influenced its quality significantly.

The saying, "It takes a village to raise a child," also comes to mind when I think of Timmy. His grandmother played an important role, as did numerous caregivers, some spending decades with him, and I would like to think that the residents of Ocean Park play their part as well. He is known, loved, and is a source of inspiration for many of us. He also defines courage.

* * *

Being the mother of a child who has medical conditions requires devotion and love. Tim's mother's experience led me to search for other people who have similar circumstances, raising a child with physical disability. By chance, I came to know Pei-Ming Sun, who lives in Indiana and is the mother of an educated son with muscular dystrophy. I am committed to share with all readers of this book the concept of "Muscular Dystrophy is not Mind Dystrophy," which I conceived in my mind after being freed from fearful and confused representations concerning people with disabilities. Pei-Ming Sun, who is active in the Muscular Dystrophy Association in Indiana and held a significant position, opened her heart and said,

> Mind and body are working together in so many ways. Unfortunately, we sometimes will have misconceptions about people who are physically disabled and judge them for their mental abilities. MD is definitely a cruel disease impacted everywhere in the body. Sadly, due to this disease, many bright young souls have to give up their dreams, hopes, and even lives. But lots of MD people I know have gotten their advanced degrees and made meaningful contributions to society. They are definitely not mind-dystrophy people. People like you and I

usually become very inspired when recognizing their beautiful minds and their strength in facing their challenges.

As I learned that Pei-Ming Sun has a deep experience with the abilities and skills that people with disabilities can share with the world, I asked her some questions:

Costa: Do you think people with muscular dystrophy get sufficient opportunity in the community to demonstrate their skills?

Pei-Ming Sun: I believe more and more people have recognized the talents and strengths of those who suffer from MD. I am not a fan of modern technology, as it creates so much e-waste for our environment, and noises for our peaceful minds. However, I have to give credit to these tools that are able to help MD patients to achieve something in their life and perhaps live independently. I cannot say we do have enough community opportunities for everyone impacted by MD. But at least, there are ways for MD people to share and communicate with the rest of society to show off their skills (computer design, books, music, drawing, writing, playing music, etc.).

Costa: Are you satisfied with the level of respect (value) that is being shown to people with muscular dystrophy? What about access to local businesses and buildings?

Pei-Ming Sun: I assume you are asking about public respect toward a person who has MD? I always respect anyone around me regardless of their physical appearance or disabilities. However, I do know that not everyone in the society is practicing what I believe in. So, I will say some people will take advantage of a person who suffers from MD, but the same person will do the same thing to others who do not have MD as well. Accessibility is always an issue for people in wheelchairs. Most cases are due to people's ignorance, not lack of respect. But I believe North America (the US and Canada) are doing a much better job compared to the rest of the world.

Costa: In a few words, what is a success story that you have experienced that benefitted someone with muscular dystrophy?

Pei-Ming Sun: Changing my perspectives about true success is the lesson I got. Naturally, I am a very ambitious and competitive person. I want to do all I can to achieve things in my life. However, being a parent of a child with DMD (the most severe and common form of MD, Duchenne muscular dystrophy), I now view true success very differently. I will say a truly successful person will work on something they have a passion for regardless of how long it will take, how difficult or lonely it can be, and how much she or he has to give up.

Having a masters degree, I had worked at a large pharmaceutical company in Indianapolis for more than eleven years. However, it became clear that working for others to get paid handsomely, but lacking the freedom and support to take care of my MD son and family, wouldn't work for me. I resigned my position, which paid me more than $80,000 a year, to become a stay-at-home mom. Of course, I have struggled financially for more than three years but I am so joyful and peaceful to be able to greet my son when he returns from school, to be right with him when he needs me at school or home, and to be able to cook homemade healthy meals to improve and maintain his overall health. And now, I have accepted a position to share my knowledge and passions to serve other MD families and patients who have struggles similar to what our family has experienced. I consider this my chance to pay it forward, as I have met so many great people in this journey. Inspired, I will do my best to live in the present, and cherish what I have.

Costa: Anything you would like to say to the world?

Pei-Ming Sun: Be positive, joyful, and thankful. Everything in life has its value in shaping who we are and providing opportunities to achieve our goals in life.

Getting to Know Tim

"Success is getting what you want;
happiness is wanting what you get."
— *Dale Carnegie, (1888-1955)*

When I heard about Tim for the first time through his mother Karen, I was taking a class called Community Healthcare and Medicaid as part of my master's studies in Public Health. I was also finishing a personal care assistance course. I was very interested to work in a field that would give me a view of community healthcare and promote my ability to understand more about how people consume healthcare services in the United States, but also to know how people with disability cope with their daily life, and community perspective toward those with physical challenges.

I had the opportunity to be connected with Tim through his mother. I met her from Craigslist, when I was looking for a job, and there I saw Tim's mom's post asking for help with her son who had MD and I was very interested in that. I decided to find out about becoming one of Tim's caregivers. I met Tim in Portland, Maine, at the company that fixes his wheelchair. I was touched to talk for the first time in my life with someone in a wheelchair, who got most of his breath from a ventilator. It was a short meeting that contributed to a new way of thinking about "Living the Present." When I left Tim, I got in my car and then took a deep breath in and let it out. In actual fact,

I had decided to work with Tim and get to know more about him.

I was scheduled for an orientation in Tim's house. It was around noon when I knocked on the door that goes directly to his living room. There are two things that everyone notices who enters Tim's living room: the number of gorgeous works of art, which are meticulously hung on the wall; and a cute curious cat named Zoey, who is either peacefully resting on a small stool near Tim's computer desk at the window sill, or running here and there.

The living room looked like a small art gallery. Some nice drawings or paintings of fish, flowers designed in different shapes, paintings of pumpkins in different colors. That day, I was touched by the art that portrayed his face in black and white. There were also some photographs that looked like they were old, but interesting.

"Welcome in," said this nice lady named Connie Johnson, whom Tim considers as his second mom. She has been providing care to Tim for a long while and has become more parent than caregiver. She was taking him from the bed to his wheelchair using the Hoyer Lift.

"Hello," Tim greeted me and smiled peacefully. I immediately noticed that he was confined to being either in bed or in a wheelchair.

The first time I saw the Hoyer Lift, I saw it in Tim's house. I was very concerned about it and wondered if I could figure out how to use it when I was going to be with him by myself.

Connie showed me how to use the Hoyer Lift with its formula of BGG (Blue-Green-Green). I kept asking about different things included in Tim's wheelchair functioning. I remember she told me, "Tim is a good teacher here; he will teach you a lot. So don't worry." When she said that, I looked at Tim and he was calmly reflecting a straightforward expression, which really created confidence inside me.

I went home after taking some notes on how to get Tim out of the bed. I asked Connie if I could come in at night to learn how to put Tim on the bed. "It's fairly the opposite of what you learned in the morning," she said. She encouraged me to come and see and let me know that Tim was going to bed at midnight.

I made a nighttime drive from Portland to Tim's house in Old Orchard Beach, a distance of nineteen miles one way. I was there a few minutes before midnight. Tim was on the computer. I didn't know exactly what he was doing. Curious, I approached to see how he was holding the mouse and the way he was navigating it. Someone from Africa like me, where there is limited affordable technological training, will think it is amazing to see someone using one hand for the computer, doing the same or better than those who have the use of two hands.

Tim was ready to go to bed. He was closing and saving some of the files containing his artwork and signing out of his Facebook and Yahoo accounts. He was doing it so very fast at that point, that I couldn't imagine how he was able to navigate the cursor with the mouse, naming the files and closing them so quickly.

When Tim is on the computer, the wheelchair has to be turned off to avoid any risk of accidentally touching the wheelchair controls, which can cause a risky sudden movement. If you forget, he will nicely remind you to turn off his wheelchair. Once the computer was turned off, the wheelchair was turned on, and Tim's right hand, which is very active while driving, was placed on the main control on the right armrest. His left hand, which he rarely uses, was placed on the left wheelchair armrest. We went into the bedroom. I was told that it's part of the routine to use the cough assist before going to bed and again in the morning after getting out of the bed. It's very helpful to clear his throat and lungs to enable free and relaxed breathing as he uses air from the ventilator. After the cough assist process, he was moved to the bed using the Hoyer Lift, which is also used to help him out of the bed.

When Tim was in bed, his cat Zoey came and stretched out on his legs and lay there, curiously looking at how her "roommate," as Tim likes calling himself, was being cared for. I noticed a visible lovely connection between Tim and Zoey.

So my shift as Tim's caregiver was scheduled to start at the beginning of the summer. That day was the first time I learned about muscular dystrophy, when I watched Tim's video posted on YouTube. "I would like to show you a very important video about myself," he told me while at the same time navigating to the YouTube search window.

Tim made the video specifically to address some of the issues he was facing in a facility in Maine. Riding his powered wheelchair, with a calm face, focusing on what he was going to do, he said to the camera, "I was diagnosed with Duchenne muscular dystrophy when I was younger, and this is a disease which progressively weakens your muscles…" (Tim's video, made in 2008, can be viewed at: http://youtu.be/VeqDruhE184)

After watching the video I let a deep breath out and felt overwhelmed to see how competently he was presenting his concerns.

Then he suggested that we could have a tour of

downtown Old Orchard Beach. I had never been there before and this was a great opportunity for me to discover the place. The Pines building where Tim lives has a lot of features for people with disabilities, especially appropriate buttons that help to go in or go out. He easily manages those doors. Using the screen board of his wheelchair, he can open up to two doors to exit or to enter the building. He told me, "Let's meet at the front door of the building." I was very concerned about letting him go, but he built my confidence and said, "Don't worry, I know how to get out from here." That was true, because I found him already outside waiting for me. He is very careful, especially when you are travelling or going somewhere with his van. He will remind you to bring the extra batteries for his ventilator. So we took two with us in the van. Getting in the van and out of the van, Tim can do himself. I only opened the door, and he drove up to the rail, until the wheelchair was locked there securely. All these things were very new to me.

We were driving along, and after a few feet Tim started giving me driving directions: "Take a left here and take the next right here," until we were in the middle of the town, close to the Atlantic Ocean. The town was very crowded and there was no place to park.

"That is very normal during summer in Old Orchard Beach (OOB)," Tim told me. "People come from all over the world to vacation here in OOB," he added.

I was wondering if we could find somewhere to park. That wasn't a concern to Tim, who is well known by many police and parking division staff from the town. One of the policemen saw us and pleasantly directed us to where there was an empty parking spot for people with disability.

I didn't know exactly where he was taking me. Many people know him. Some of them came and gave him a hug, others a kiss on the cheek. From the other side of the road I could hear and see people shouting, "Hi Tim!" and waving.

I realized that he is very popular in OOB. He was leading our tour and I was blindly following. Soon, we were in a place with thousands of people. I remember the place was very loud. On the left, music, on the right Karaoke, and in front of us there was a bar with a band. Many things were going on there. The place is called the Pier. Some grownups who didn't know Tim were looking at him with kindhearted expressions, and their young children looked with a sense of strangeness at this person in a wheelchair. At the same time, many people who knew him were friendly, approaching Tim and talking to him. They all had a common question they were asking Tim: "Are you doing any art these days? Do you have an art show coming up?" And he responded that he had been doing a lot of art to prepare for the show that was going to happen on July 4th, 2011. I began to realize that Tim is an amazing man. Many people know him as a professional artist. We spent almost three hours going from one place to another, before ending up in a Thai restaurant where he had something to eat.

We went back to his apartment around 10:00 pm. He went directly to the computer. I requested of him that he go directly to bed. Tim resisted and said that he had many tasks to do in order to be ready for the art show in which he was planning to participate.

The night was fruitful, as he was able to finish some of the wonderful drawings he made. He then printed fish and flowers that he digitally drew, and I helped him to put them in picture frames. "I like what I did and I am now ready to go to bed," he told me. My heart was full of joy for the achievements he could do with a committed heart.

* * *

Caring for our health is another factor that is important to a mindful way of living and we can make good choices when we focus on the ability to do so.

"Costa," Tim said to me when I visited him at his apartment, "I watched a show of a man who spent more than sixty days drinking just juice that he was making by himself,"

He could not tell me more about the show, but he knew exactly what he wanted to do. At the same time he was searching online through many stores to find the cost of a juice maker.

"Costa, can we go somewhere?" Tim patiently asked me.

I said, "Yes, certainly."

Smiling, he asked, "Can you turn my wheelchair on and move my right hand to the joy stick?" The wheelchair was switched on and his hand was put on the remote, and he was ready to go. We got in the van and he asked me if we could visit the Target store, seven to ten minutes from where he lives.

While entering the store, we saw a lady smoking near a little child in a stroller. I asked Tim what we could do to save that child from being a victim of cigarette smoke. I told him that I recently had a similar experience with someone who was indifferently smoking too close to her child. With some hesitation, he told me that we should approach the lady and tell her that it is not good to smoke around the child.

While we were in the store parking lot, I saw one of the store employees talking with the lady who was smoking around her own child. I approached her and said, "Can you please go and advise that lady you were talking with to stop smoking around the baby and kindly advise her that the baby does not deserve to be around any kind of smoke?" She promised to tell her what we wished.

When we got inside the store, Tim asked me if we could find a store assistant. I hurried away and found one.

"Can you tell us where to find a juice maker?" he asked. The store assistant's mind could not understand at first what Tim was asking, and she turned to look at me and asked me, "What do you guys want?"

"Tim knows what he wants and he can repeat that for you," I said. He jumped right in and said clearly, "I would like to look at a juice maker."

That entire exchange is typical of how a lot of people react to seeing someone like Tim in a wheelchair. He has a clear speaking voice, yet I have experienced a number of times that he will ask for something in a store and the cashier or assistant will turn and look at me. I think the reason this happens is that, when we are predisposed to not understand, we cannot understand. Seeing him in his wheelchair getting his breath by sipping through a mouthpiece attached to an oxygen ventilator—even though he speaks clearly—people assume that this wheelchair-bound person's ability to talk or to clearly express what he wants must also be impaired. What we believe is what our minds sometimes falsely interpret. When we see past our conditioning, we are ready to recognize an ability in someone like Tim—then understanding comes easily.

We found where the juice makers were displayed and he chose one. It was almost 10:00 pm, but still he was determined to make some juice before going to sleep.

"I want to undertake a new healthy diet system," he said to me. "Do you think we can go to Hannaford and buy some fruits there? I think they close at 11:00 pm!" So we left the Target store and went to Hannaford, his favorite store.

When Tim sets up a goal, he will not rest until he achieves it. His goal that day was to make juice with his new juicer and start the diet he learned about from a TV show, in order to experience how someone can feel healthier from juice that he makes for himself. "This does not mean that I will not be eating other food, but I want to change my eating behavior and focus on homemade juice," he said, as we drove to the Hannaford in Saco.

We did some quick shopping while the store was closing its doors. We filled the cart with the items to purchase. Tim knows some foods that even the cashiers could not figure out. A white root called daikon could not be found in the register. He tried to explain, and spelled its name for the cashier, but in vain. After a few more minutes spent on unsuccessfully trying to figure out the cost of the item, the cashier decided to give it to him for free!

We arrived home after 11:00 p.m. and Tim still wanted to make some juice. "Are you okay if we can juice something quickly?" he anxiously requested of me, at the same time looking at the clock hanging on the kitchen wall. I know all about Tim's commitment and I could not resist or even reason with him about the time.

I asked him what he wanted to juice, he said, "Just fruits." We set up the new juice maker and started to juice oranges, pineapples, bananas, grapes, and strawberries. We soon had a good quantity of juice. Bright people are always known for their curiosity, and while I was juicing, Tim was navigating his wheelchair around and thinking at the same time.

New experiments in juicing came about. "Can you help to juice some more things?" he asked me. I asked him what else apart from fruits. Tim said, "How about juicing some broccoli, kale, a little bit of green beans, some ginger, sweet potatoes, spinach, and tomatoes?" I was laughing about preparing such an odd mixture of vegetables.

When I was chopping tomatoes, I almost cut my finger and Tim, who likes joking, warned me, "Pay attention and make sure we do not have finger juice." I could not keep from laughing.

All right, the juice was ready! As he was testing, he found he did not like the vegetable juice we had made, especially the taste of the kale, which dominated all of the other flavors. He decided he could not discard it, and instead decided to keep it in the fridge for the next day.

A few days later while enjoying the juice diet, Tim added more challenging and interesting ideas on what to juice. One evening, we spent three hours juicing, but one thing, which he decided to add, killed all of the other flavors. That was the hot jalapeño pepper.

"I would like to add one jalapeño and see how the taste will be," he said with confidence. The jalapeño did not respond positively to his wish and the result was very spicy, which led to the failure of our juicing that night. "Let's put that in the fridge and I will try to mix it with other stuff tomorrow," he said. What a night!

* * *

Looking into the living room from the kitchen where we were juicing, we were surprised that we didn't see Tim's cat Zoey anywhere.

"Where is the kitty?" Tim asked, moving around with his wheelchair.

He realized that the front door was open and told me that he was pretty sure that Zoey had gone outside. I went outside and looked around. I could not see Zoey.

It was already 11:00 p.m. and Tim was afraid that his lovely friend Zoey was going to be killed by foxes. I grabbed a flashlight and went around in the bushes to see if I could find the cat. By chance, I found Zoey enjoying the darkness of the bush. She ran back inside Tim's house. Tim, the man who likes joking, asked Zoey, "How was the vacation you are coming back from?" There was a relieved happiness in Tim's face.

Whose Business?

In Tim's Words

I always get into questioning my mind when Costa asks me about "whose business." I like that and it teaches me to think a lot about my health choices.

I have a regular routine of having cough assists that help to keep my lungs clear. My caregivers help me to have a cough assist at least two to four times a day.

Costa sometimes calls me "magic head." This came about when once he happened to forget to give me my pills, and before I slept I reminded him that I hadn't taken them. This happened two more times. Costa calls me "magic head" because I have a very good memory!

I do respect advice: My caregivers have been helping me a lot with my health. I like that kind of advice, though sometimes I feel confused, especially when I fail to put into practice some of the good advice I have been given. My caregivers contribute a lot to my life. Costa posts health-related articles on my Facebook wall about the many ways to maintain the body's health. The article Costa sent to me on the importance of sleeping before midnight and waking up before 9:00 a.m. helped me change my sleeping behavior. Sometimes I sleep too late for no reason. When I first read the article, I took it as an attack on me and my mind. That is why I told Costa that sometimes I am confused. However, with time, I understood that "it is my business to sleep on time and wake up on time." So thank you, Costa.

Tim's Religious Beliefs

The first night I spent in Tim's house I was very surprised. When Tim was ready to sleep, he gently asked, "Costa, I heard you are a Christian. Can I pray for you before we both sleep?" I was full of joy and welcomed his wish. He prayed for me and I did the same for him.

On the wall in Tim's room, right in front of his bed, there is a picture that portrays Jesus raising his hand and providing blessings. This picture is strategically placed on the wall so Tim can see it every time he goes to bed. The text says, "Eternal Father, I offer You the Body and Blood, Soul and Divinity of Your Dearly Beloved Son, Our Lord, Jesus Christ, in atonement for our sins and those of the whole world. For the sake of His Passion, have mercy on us and on the whole world, Holy God, Holy Mighty One, Holy Immortal." I was very curious and asked Tim why he had that picture there.

He said, "This prayer always makes me know that God is with me and he forgives me. I do believe that God has done many things for me and that is why I still breathe today; God loves me. I didn't make up this prayer. One time I went to pray at the cathedral in Portland, and we started with the rosaries and that part really touched me." Tim added, "I went also to the Saint Margarets in Old Orchard Beach and during the rosaries I was again touched with that part of the prayer and decided to print it on paper and display it so that I can see it every night when I go to bed."

Tim believes that everyone has a right to pray in his

or her own way. "I feel blessed when I go to my church, St. Joseph Church in Biddeford, or to downtown Saco, to Most Holy Trinity Church, where I had my first communion, or to the First Parish Congregational Church-UCC in downtown Saco. I like the way I pray," he calmly said.

One evening I received a Facebook message from Tim's mom telling me that she had registered Tim for a three-day spiritual retreat at the Marie Joseph Spiritual Center in Biddeford Pool. The spiritual retreat was also about watercolor painting.

We were a little bit late getting there. When we entered the room, Tim was a little flustered and said, "I am the only man here." That was true, and he looked shy. He approached the table anyway and welcomed the retreat in his mind. As he cannot hold a paintbrush, he was compelled to use his computer. I was amazed that, within a few minutes, you could see on his computer screen that he had painted an elegant sky.

After that evening session we went back home. Tim could not sleep there because of his physical needs, which require specific conditions, including a special bed and ventilator that are not found everywhere. On the road going home, he told me, "When I entered the room, I wondered why my mother registered me in that spiritual workshop, when I was the only man there, but later I realized that I should focus on the workshop." The same night, his mother called him and wanted to know how the session went.

Tim replied, "I was very shy and wondered why you wanted me to be in that workshop as the only man, but then I enjoyed it." His mother laughed. Tim said to me, "I like going to places that can help me to think about

God." Arriving home, he told me that he would like to use the computer a little. I realized a spiritual revival was in his mind. He went to a certain window and started interpreting the song "The Stand."

> You stood before creation
> Eternity within Your hand
> You spoke the earth into motion
> My soul now to stand
>
> You stood before my failure
> Carried the Cross for my shame
> My sin weighed upon Your shoulders
> My soul now to stand
>
> So what can I say
> What can I do
> But offer this heart O God
> Completely to You
>
> So I'll walk upon salvation
> Your Spirit alive in me
> This life to declare Your promise
> My soul now to stand
>
> So what can I say
> What can I do
> But offer this heart O God
> Completely to You
>
> So I'll stand
> With arms high and heart abandoned
> In awe of the One who gave it all
>
> So I'll stand
> My soul Lord to You surrendered
> All I am is Yours

When he was done, he called to me and said, "Costa, this is my favorite song and I like the way it inspires me." After that, he played it on YouTube and told me to leave the computer open while I was assisting him with the transfer to the bed. When on his bed ready to sleep, Tim said to me, "Costa, Let us pray."

We prayed and he told me, "Costa, I do believe your idea where you like saying that we are much more the spirit than the body, because both grieving and happiness are more parts of our thinking than our body." I told him that whatever happens to us, grieving or happiness is an echo of our mind.

More Experiences with Tim

The moon shows its shining face indiscriminately. Both those who are struggling with their fear and those who find their pathways of peace enjoy the luminous light from the moon.

The moon's smile does not last for long, but it is a long time changing. Its full appearance happens only a few days every month and provides a sense of love that everyone needs to live and to share.

Tim will not miss an occasion to see the full moon.

One evening he said, "Costa, I would like to drive by the beach to see the appearance of the full moon rising." We grabbed the camera and drove to the beach. It was too cold and at first we watched the moon through the windshield of his van. Then I ran quickly to the ocean and shot some video of the moon's reflections on the ocean. "I like watching the full moon," he said. "It brings peace inside myself. It relaxes my mind."

* * *

Halloween: Imagine seeing Tim celebrate this spooky event! In 2013 on a late October night, he told me that he was very excited to be participating in a Halloween event that was organized by one of the well-known restaurant-bars in southern Maine called *Jimmy The Greek's*. I asked him why he chose that place. He said, "People are nice there and I know a lot of them. One day the owner invited me to the microphone, which was a big honor for me. It is also close to where I live here in Old Orchard Beach," he added.

What happened? Tim did not make it. That Saturday was the nastiest weather. Snow—yes, snow in October! Snow fell all evening and Tim decided to remain home. The freak storm set records in Maine as the largest single snowfall in October.

"I felt so bad to miss that event, but I had a fun time here at home," he told me when I came to his house a few nights later. "Look at this picture on my Facebook page." He was pointing his cursor at his Facebook profile picture. I yelled! It was so funny and spooky to look at. Tim's face was made up with big dark circles around his eyes, pale white skin with red veins spider over his face, and a jagged black scar across his neck. He told me that one of the lovely nurses who takes care of him did that for him. I nearly fell over laughing. He truly looked scary.

"I am so glad to see I have participated in this event," Tim said. "I like having fun like that sometimes," he added. I told him that we don't have Halloween in my country, Rwanda, and even where I was born in Burundi and where I grew up in the Democratic Republic of Congo, I had never seen people celebrating anything like Halloween.

We spent some time together looking on the Internet at how people celebrate Halloween.

* * *

Christmas: "It is time to think about my friends and my caregivers and which gifts I will get for them," said Tim. The plan was set at the end of November. Together with his second mother, Connie, he started working diligently on selecting gifts, tagging the packages, as well as decorating the house.

Tim is a Christian and believes in Jesus Christ as his Savior and Redeemer. "It's my right to believe in Jesus Christ as my Savior," he said.

He loves Christmas Eve. "I am excited to go down to Connecticut during Christmas and will spend some time with my mother and then go on some tours of New York," he said. "It's nice to celebrate Christmas Eve because it is all about my salvation," he said. He added that he thanks his mother for having thought about that for him.

He told me that he likes to celebrate many of these important events, as part of his participation as a person in this world.

* * *

One evening Tim and I had to evacuate his apartment for aeration for at least two hours, while the apartment was treated to combat fleas. I asked him, "Where do you think we can go hang out?" He had a good idea.

"Can we go to the conference room within the Pines?

I can sit there with my computer and I can do my home-work," he tranquilly told me. As usual, he quickly added, "What do you think?" I replied that I was comfortable with that.

We went to the conference room and at first look you could see a nice table surrounded with gorgeous red chairs. Tim jokingly told me, "I am going to chair the conference and that is why I have to sit at the front in the main chair of the table." Tim likes developing imaginative scenes that can attract your attention and focus on the interaction you both are sharing. I told him that I had never seen a confer-ence with two people. He quickly jumped in saying, "Oh, others are coming, although they are late." He was joking again.

The computer was set up on the table and Tim was looking forward to doing the homework for his online course, Introduction to Astronomy, sitting in the leader's chair. That's when we discovered there wasn't any Internet wireless connection. He told me that the conference room didn't have a wireless network. I was little a bit disap-pointed. Tim, however, was not discouraged.

"It's okay," he said, smiling. Even though he would not be connected to the Internet on the brand new laptop his mom had just bought for him. We were both busy. I was benefiting from that peaceful moment to review my GRE (Graduate Record Exam) book, since I would have to take that exam for graduate studies purposes.

Tim's spirit is full of creativity and I am not exag-gerating when I say that his mind has thousands of art dreams. In a short time, he had drawn a dazzling blue sky, while at the same time playing cards. It was hard for me to understand how his mind could focus on doing multiple things at the same time. All the time, ideas flow from his mind and he does these things easily. We spent almost three hours there, and then he told me that he wanted to go back to the apartment.

I packed up some things and made a few trips carrying them out to the van, then returned to help him with opening the door. When I went back to the room where he was sitting, he looked at me shyly and smiled. I approached him, curious to know why he looked so shy and happy at the same time. He said, "I wrote something about my girlfriend. Let me read it for you:"

> My Dear, you are so amazing. You make me very happy. I can't wait till I see you in person again. You're like an angel from heaven. You're someone whom I've been looking for my whole life. Your smile brightens me up. I pray that we can be together to love each other, to cherish each other, and share true happiness forever.
>
> I dreamt I kissed you. I leaned over then just got close and kissed you. Then you told me you love me and I said, "you love me" in joy, then I said, "I love you. I am so glad you love me. I feel so happy and whole."

Limitations

The able-bodied constantly and without thought take a lot of things for granted in this world. Travelling around, driving cars, navigating sidewalks, accessing places like beaches, restaurants, and other public facilities with ease. I hope that when seeing a wheelchair-bound person in public, able-bodied people are reminded to feel grateful for their able-bodiedness, and feel less like complaining about difficulties in their own lives.

While people with muscular dystrophy don't put limitations on themselves, the environment does limit their access to many public services that others take advantage of without thinking twice.

Many old buildings were built without thinking about people in wheelchairs. We will not spend time wondering about the reasons why building owners or architects were not considering this matter, but instead, focus on how innovation can be used to help people in wheelchairs to access these premises.

But we can all wonder why there are new buildings built without wheelchair facilities. What would you think if this happened to you? You really want to go to a new restaurant and yet you will not be able to enjoy the place and their foods just because the restaurant is not wheelchair accessible.

Tim's birthday is November 8th, and in 2011 he was going to be twenty-eight. I was not available to celebrate that birthday with him. I was in Los Angeles attending an AIDS walk. However, I promised Tim that on the evening of November 18th I would take him to dinner and I left to him the choice of a good restaurant he wanted to visit. He chose a new restaurant in Portland.

We drove to Portland from his home in Old Orchard Beach. We knew where the restaurant was, but we didn't know that his access to it would be limited. We parked his van off the street and followed the sidewalk for a good five minutes. When we got to the restaurant, we were met by a challenging situation. Tim couldn't get in, because the restaurant didn't have an access path for wheelchairs. Tim was little a bit frustrated and started to give some unfeasible suggestions. "Can you lay those two restaurant standing signs down and I can drive over them to get in the restaurant?" Tim asked. The lady who was restaurant manager was apologetic, saying, "Sorry, sorry, sorry, let's see what we can do." She called some of her stronger staff persons and suggested lifting up Tim's wheelchair with Tim in it, which was quite impossible. Tim is wheelchair bound; so you'd have to lift both the wheelchair and Tim. I had already experienced that even if Tim is on his bed and not in the wheelchair, that his empty wheelchair is difficult to push. It is very heavy. Furthermore it would be very risky to lift Tim and the wheelchair together. I resisted that idea and told the lady that it should be a lesson for them to remember, that the restaurant should be able to be visited by both able-bodied people and people in wheelchairs. Fortunately, Tim had chosen a second alternative restaurant nearby, where we then enjoyed his birthday dinner.

* * *

Springtime 2012 brought surprising weather. Tuesday, April 17, around 5:00 p.m., it was above 75 degrees Fahrenheit, and Tim wished to drive his wheelchair around and see how the beach looked and enjoy the unusually warm weather. I was with him and we walked under the beautiful pine trees of Ocean Park breathing nice oxygen-filled fresh air. We approached the beach and the beach area. We could see some people waving to Tim enthusiastically, and those who knew him stopped to say hi. Between the road near the beach and the beach itself we saw a long wooden ramp. Tim was very eager to drive his wheelchair on it so that he could at least see the beach at a closer view. But the wooden path would not let him do so due to the heaviness of his wheelchair. Some of the wooden path was already broken in several places. He tried anyway and unfortunately got his wheelchair stuck. I helped to push a little bit, and he managed to free himself, and we got off of the wooden path.

We continued our drive and walk around the Ocean Park, until Tim decided that it was time for us to go back home.

On our way back, he told me that he would like to have big tires on his wheelchair that would help him to freely drive on the sands. "That would be expensive I guess," he said. Once home, he told me that he had to do his philosophy homework and added that he already had a subject. I asked him what the subject was. He responded, "Why can people in wheelchairs not access the Old Orchard Beach? I feel like I would wish one day for that beach to completely offer access to all people without any difficulty."

* * *

While many organizations are committed to access for all, some of the educational institutions and resource centers are still challenges for those with a disability. Inadequate materials for people with a disability limit their ability to learn and practice what they've learned.

One night Tim had to go to the star field observatory center near Kennebunk to identify constellations and other objects in space as part of the assignment he had in the online Introduction to Astronomy class he was taking. He had two days of intense reviews and studying for what he was going to observe at the center. The instructor told Tim that evening time around six was the most appropriate time to do that observation. I drove him to the center and made sure we were there before six so that we didn't miss seeing the planet Jupiter.

We drove down from Old Orchard Beach to Kennebunk and were a little bit late, but the instructor was there to welcome us.

The place was muddy and it was very chilly. There was no electricity at the center and it was very dark. We were compelled to use the van lights for him to see to drive his wheelchair to the telescope that was pointed to where Jupiter was supposed to pass. But the soil was very wet and the wheelchair repeatedly got stuck in the mud. The instructor and I had to push and push, trying to see if Tim could position himself at the telescope and experience what he had been learning.

Unfortunately, regrettably, unluckily, Tim couldn't reach the telescope's ocular to observe the sky. He must, by any means, report on what he saw from the field. His chair could easily recline backward and so he observed with his own eyes. Despite challenges that prevented him from looking through the telescope, he could still identify some galaxies, and proved that he knows what he learned.

The instructor was really happy for the attention that Tim was putting on the sky observation, though you could see from his eyes a sorry expression for the lack of access to the telescope for Tim. The weather was really cold and it is much advised for people with muscular dystrophy to not be exposed to cold weather. But there was still some useful data that Tim wanted and he couldn't get it without looking through the telescope.

Tim asked the instructor if I could look on his behalf and he could interpret the findings. Having compassion, the instructor accepted.

I wanted to get Tim out of the cold as soon as possible. I rushed to drive his van closer so that he could get in. But his wheelchair was stuck in the mud. The instructor and I again pushed it and at the same time Tim accelerated hard, and finally the wheelchair reached the van ramp. He got into the van and out of the cold.

I started looking through the telescope and wrote down what I observed. I saw for the first time the planet Jupiter with its moons and felt challenged in my heart by the fact that Tim, who was taking that class, was totally unable to see it, not only because he has muscular dystrophy, but also because the telescope was not made to be accessible for people like him.

I wrote down everything. Tim managed to interpret all the data I collected and compiled his assignment. What I realized in the field was that I was awed even more than before by Tim, who takes it easy with what he faces all the time. He was really peaceful and enjoyed the experience for what it was.

I asked him to talk about challenges he faces in his daily life. "My life is now full of perseverance," he said.

* * *

One night around midnight as I helped Tim to get ready for bed, and after setting the oxygen mask and chinstrap on his face, I asked him if I could ask him some questions.

"Oh yeah!" he said. "I can't sleep for one hour or even more since it's my time to think about what I can do to create and design facilities for people with muscular dystrophy."

I got out my recording device and reminded him of some of the sorrowful moments I had with him and that I wanted to hear his comments. He looked at me attentively. I told him that one sorrowful moment that really touched me was when he couldn't get into the restaurant and instead, he peacefully enjoyed the dinner offered to him in the second restaurant on his twenty-eighth birthday; and another was when he couldn't look in the telescope and enjoy the galaxy, as part of his assignment.

Costa: "As someone with muscular dystrophy, what were your feelings when those things happened to you?"

Tim: Having muscular dystrophy shouldn't be a barrier for learning or accessing public places. I do understand when I can't visit my relatives, friends, or even your family, Costa my friend. Some of these families and friends don't own the houses they live in and they don't have the rights or choices to put ramps. No choice. Saying no choice isn't only limiting to those friends and relatives who can't do anything to the buildings they are renting, but also to me. What can I do? I sometimes take a moment and think on how we people with muscular dystrophy are limited in too many things and how some people ignore us and our needs. It's okay, that is the way we are, but government, organizations, and even communities, can do something to allow us to live limitlessly.

When I went to the field tour in Kennebunk for my astronomy class, I didn't know that I would find it challenging to look through the telescope. As you realized, I tried to recline my wheelchair in all directions so that I could position myself straight to the telescope oculars but all those efforts were in vain. And I am really sorry, I shouldn't have kept you all that time outside in that nippy weather like that. I think there must be some telescopes appropriate for people who are wheelchair bound like me. They might be expensive or rare to find in our area. I can't pretend that I wasn't sad; I was, and went away sad, since I didn't have any alternative.

That star field observatory center in Kennebunk is not as much visited as restaurants. It was very strange to me when we couldn't get in that restaurant situated in one of the most popular streets of the state of Maine. The restaurant itself is ranked among the top five best restaurants in Portland, but without easy access for people who are wheelchair bound. What can you say or think about that? I am not ashamed. Rather, they should be ashamed.

I have been going to different restaurants and that day was a special one to me. It was an exceptional offer that you planned for a long time to give me for my birthday. I chose that restaurant after I critically balanced it out among others because I had never been there. I didn't even have the courage to call and ask if the restaurant was wheelchair accessible simply because I trusted that it should be due to its good standing. I tried my best to give them some suggestions but, as you experienced, I couldn't get in. Putting a ramp at such a restaurant can't at all cost them a lot, but the problem is in understanding the value of people with disability. You can ask yourself why that restaurant is not wheelchair accessible and another one is?

There are still many public places that don't give easy access or access at all to people in wheelchairs. I have in my mind two particular public places that I think about all the time, because they limit my access to important learning experiences, and enjoyment of local attractions.

The first one is the painting room at my school, the University of Southern Maine. I have been a student at that university for more than two years now, but unfortunately, I can't access the painting room. As an artist, I frequently wish to visit that room but I really can't get in. I wished I could register for painting class but I couldn't really do that since that painting room doesn't have facilities for individuals in wheelchairs. And yet, this is a university, which hosts all groups of people without any kind of discrimination. One day I was joking with my mother, who wished as well that I could take painting class, that I could sue that university. My caregivers are always surprised when they go along with me to the school and find that there is a place I can't really access, simply because I can't walk.

The second public place is the beach. I have lived here in Old Orchard Beach for a long time and I don't have any plans to live elsewhere. This is my hometown along the Atlantic coast in southern Maine. During summer, this town hosts hundreds of thousands of tourists coming from different parts of the world, attracted by this beautiful and popular beach in Maine. I believe I am not wrong to say that the beach in the town of Old Orchard Beach is among the most gorgeous beaches in the USA.

Unfortunately, I can't go onto the beach because I am wheelchair bound. I like going on the paved road that goes downtown to see new faces and the huge numbers of guests, and I feel like I am the only one who is not allowed to reach the beach.

That beach belongs to all of us and is cared for by the government. That means there must be a way that wheelchair access can be added, but what's missing is the value that people in wheelchairs deserve.

So, everyone has the ability to access the beach except me, and those with physical challenges like me. Whose fault do you think that is? I can't change my body, but the beach can be modified to provide easy access to everybody.

The town can do something simple, like putting a small platform with a ramp that can help a wheelchair to travel over it. We can be alerted to not visit the beach when there is a windy forecast so that we won't be blown away by the water. I am pretty sure it won't disfigure the beauty of the beach. I have heard there are some wheelchairs that can go on the sand but they must be too expensive for my mother to afford.

It is time for each and every one to open their hearts and allow people with disabilities to be fully integrated into our society. This cannot be achieved until we find ourselves with a peaceful mind. It is very hard when I am not peaceful, to value others. I hope the town officials, university directors, and others who have the spaces that aren't wheelchair accessible will read this book and develop strategies that show love and respect to everyone."

Accessibility does not mean only the ability of being here and there easily but also accessing all the opportunities that the so called, "able-people" have. If we take at least one second to put ourselves in the shoes of those with muscular dystrophy we can understand how all of us are one, and see the need to treat and to be treated equally.

* * *

There are many institutions that put in their daily programs the access-for-all consideration. A good example to follow is that of the Unitarian Universalist churches and Methodist churches who consider accessibility as "a theological issue." I was really touched when I read their article, "Accessibility Information for Unitarian Universalist Churches." A lovingly created interfaith publication written collaboratively for the United Methodist Church and the Unitarian Universalist Association Published in 2010" (www.uua.org/documents/idbm/accessibility/manual.pdf), with vital principles that everyone can bear in mind to help make this world an nondiscriminating one. The three principles state:

—"Our congregation believes that all people, including people with disabilities, are valued as individuals, having inherent worth and dignity."

—"Our congregation encourages people, with and without disabilities, to practice their faith and use their gifts in worship, service, study, and leadership."

—"Our congregation is making an effort to remove barriers of architecture, communications and attitudes that exclude people with disabilities from full and active participation."

If we can all value these principles and apply them in different organizations, all people with disabilities can finally gain the ground where they can share their skills that we think are limited.

My lovely friend Tim had the courage to apply for a temporary position to teach young kids at a summer camp. The organizers trusted Tim's skills and gave him an opportunity to show his ability to transfer his knowledge. He happily taught the kids how to do digital arts. It was so encouraging to see how the camp organizers provided credit to Tim without focusing on his physical aspects, but rather on what he could do.

Spiritual Surprises

On Friday, December 2, 2011, Tim told me that he would like to go the cathedral in Portland for the evening mass. We got into his van and he said that he would like to drive by his old house, which was taken down because they wanted to build another house.

It was around 6:30 p.m. and very dark, as it was winter. There was another car coming behind us with glaring headlights and I said to Tim, "Let this guy pass so that we can see where to stop where your house will be built." When we stopped for the car to pass, it came and stopped parallel to us. It was Tim's mother! He said, "I was expecting you in Connecticut, not in Maine!" His mother came and got in the van and asked us where we were going. Tim said, "I want to see how our old house was demolished and then I want to go to the cathedral in Portland to pray." His mother was astonished and said, "I came here to the house for the same reason, and then I'm going to a retreat in Biddeford Pool." I told them that they are really connected by spirit, since they planned the same things at the same time. We visited the house and then went to the cathedral in Portland. The evening mass headed by Bishop Richard J. Malone was very devout. It was accompanied by the wonderful spiritual music of the *Cathedral Capella Musica* directed by Leon Griesbach. When we were on the way to the cathedral, Tim told me that I would be inspired by the nice voices of the choir.

Tim loves God. He believes that God can handle the hard projects of life. I remembered when he was praying before sleeping, and he said, "God forgive me, give me love and strength." He never thinks that it is difficult for someone with muscular dystrophy to have a girlfriend. Rather he said, "God has the ability to show and to bring someone into a relationship with you."

Every day I weep in joy
(A Poem by Tim)

Every day I weep in joy about what you have done
    for us
Every day I weep when I feel your love
I weep in joy to be counted among your flock
I chose to avoid the lonely dark evil "nothingness
    prison"
So Every day I weep in joy
I cry,
I mourn,
Not the death or the loss of our transient earthly
    body
but the loss of souls to hell
dying lost
descended
thrown fast and hard
you lay in the fetal position
no motion
no light
aloneness
pain
misery
agony
family friends lost

never will they return
you will long for their embrace
This will not last a hundred years
This will not last a thousand years
This will not last a million years
or 1 billion years
But forever
You will beg
You will scream
No one will hear you
You will feel this pain
Physically
Mentally
Emotionally
Spiritually
Not like you do on Earth
This pain will be magnified beyond all measurable
    degrees forever.
Every day I weep in joy.

* * *

One summer evening, Tim said that he would like to go with me to a concert at the Salvation Army in Old Orchard Beach. I told him that I would like that too. We drove there and found hundreds of people queuing for the concert. I didn't know who the artist was and how famous he might be to attract such a big number of people. Tim knew everything, and he calmly told me when we were in the line that I did know one of his songs.

"You like listening to his song on the computer, Costa," he said gently.

The queue was very long and some people were trying to show their compassion toward Tim and me so that we could go ahead to present our tickets without standing too long in line. One of the volunteers came to ask us if we would like to go straight to the kiosk to present our tickets.

"What do you think, Costa?" he asked.

I told him that I was fine to be in line. He suggested that we could wait. I told the volunteer that we were fine waiting in line and I thanked her for her bigheartedness.

I didn't know that Tim had some extra tickets to donate for people who could not afford to buy them. When we arrived at the kiosk, he gave two tickets to the cashier and said, "Can you give these extra two tickets to somebody who may need them?" My heart was touched that he had thought about other people in need when he got those tickets.

We finally got to the concert seating. A volunteer came and guided us to the front. The artist was Mark Schultz, a famous gospel singer from Nashville, Tennessee. I could not remember his song until he sang, "Love has come," which brought joy and tears to many people. When the artist finished the song, Tim asked me if I remembered it, and I said yes.

You notice Tim's positive mindfulness when you are a friend of his on Facebook, where he always encourages his friends with muscular dystrophy to have hope of being, to live optimistically and focus on their abilities to do things and be thankful to God for everything, especially when they present some hopeless ideas.

Education

Studying requires courage and perseverance. It can be a challenging journey, with many hills and valleys. When you hear stories from different people with muscular dystrophy, one thing you may notice is that they are well educated and informed. Many are in school, while others have already finished their education.

If you are in Tim's house, take one of the artworks that are in his living room and look closely at it. You will see the signature, "Timothy Stoklosa." Tim is a prolific artist. He is always learning and creating more and his success comes from being a good student with a positive attitude.

"I like to think of each step as an easy one, and then I will go with it successfully," he told me.

It's very interesting to be with him when he is so quiet, working on his homework on the computer, focusing on some artwork, or even refreshing his mind with a Scrabble game. He pauses when he wants some help with using the bathroom or, having some water to drink.

I remember this wonderful moment: Tim and I were in the apartment and you could hear only the refrigerator sounds from the kitchen and his ventilator that supplements his breathing. No one was talking; he was very concentrated on his homework.

"Look at this Costa!" he said, after four hours of serenely focusing on his astronomy online class. He maximized the homework and got 20 out of 20. I got goose bumps, and tears in my eyes looking at him.

"You are so amazing Tim," I told him earnestly.

"Thank you," he said.

That was something special, since only a few times on a final test, he had scored 92 percent. Children may be "breastfed" various attitudes from their parents. I am saying this because Tim's mother is a CPA and a talented lady. She successfully studies philosophy and English; and she is confident that her son has the full ability to study.

Tim is a good example to help relieve all of the mind's confusions toward people with muscular dystrophy, especially in the academic field. He studies attentively and courageously. He is a serious student and is able to put into action what he has learned.

Commitment is a simple adventure.

It is very hard for people who don't know Tim to envision the picture of him as someone who goes to school, unless you spend some time with him. However, his commitment and love of academics are real. An anonymous philosopher wrote: "The happiest people don't necessarily have the best of everything; they just make the best of everything they have." Every day is a new discovery for him. His creativity changes and improves with every sunrise.

When we started writing this book, Tim was taking two classes, Multimedia, which was an in-class course, and Introduction to Astronomy, an online class.

As part of the multimedia class, Tim wanted to video some things and post them on the school's Blackboard (the school's online interactive system that enables colleagues to see each other's work). It was around 5:30 p.m. and I wondered how the video was going to be done.

"I am going to be a film director," he told me. It was kind of nippy outside, but he made sure he was warmly dressed. Apart from not having the physical ability to put on clothes by himself, he has a practical knowledge of what is important. A few words allowed him to be well protected from the cold weather. "Can I put on my black jacket? Can I put on my black hat and that black scarf around my neck?" were his requests. We went outside the building and started recording the trees and the bushes around the building. "Can you video me entering the van?" he asked. I ran and opened the sliding door of the van and the ramp that allows him to drive into the van, and videoed his movement. That wasn't enough for him. He thought that people might be worried to see him in the van without any protection from all the movement that occurs while driving.

"Can you video my wheelchair lock?" he requested. I did, and he explained how the lock installed in his van fastens the wheelchair so it can't move.

What next? "I want to video the road around the town of Old Orchard Beach while we are driving. Can we video that please?" he asked. I was very skeptical about how I could hold a video camera while driving. At the same time, I didn't want him to miss those shots, as he wanted to post them the same night as part of his multimedia class assignment. We were careful and, praise the Lord, we did it peacefully. I warned him that we shouldn't do chancy things like that again. "I am sorry," he responded, some-what sheepishly.

Tim likes joking, and I remember one day I asked him where he got that joking aptitude. "From my daddy," he responded. While we were videoing, we passed through a cemetery in Saco, the town next to where Tim lives in Old Orchard Beach. He told me that he did not want to miss some video shots of the cemetery. We backed up and drove into the graveyard and started to shoot some video there. We could not get good pictures since it was really dark and we could only see where the van lights were projecting.

While we were exiting the cemetery, Tim said, "It's very sad that we didn't see any Zombies." I couldn't get my breath as I laughed and laughed. Good comedians rarely get such a laugh. His delivery was perfectly timed. While I was laughing, he was very calmly watching my reaction to his joke. When I asked him if he had ever seen Zombies, he responded deadpan, "They don't exist."

In the World

While expanding the new discovery of perceptions toward people with physical attributes, I started seeing that people with physical disability are brilliant at doing many things, especially giving value to the opportunity of learning and creating. There are still many people who equate the physical disability observation to life inability: "She is using a walker to walk so that must mean she can't do anything useful." Everyone has an example in the workplace or in the community where a tremendous kind of discrimination is aimed at people with a disability.

In North America and in other developed countries, a good number of people with physical disability attend school, though at a certain point the choice for education fields is limited by the low status they experience in society. They study with no hope of finding a job.

In most of the countries in Africa, people with a disability have a low or non-existent social status. They are seen as having nothing to contribute to the society. It is believed that people with disability are totally dependent; that they are also mentally limited, and that their minds think in a different way.

* * *

As my thinking became clearer and clearer regarding those with physical disability, I committed to explore in different parts of the world how people with physical disabilities overcome their fear and find a successful way of living by adopting a positive lifestyle, which can be a lesson to all of us. With this change in my awareness, I was freed to see this truth and became friends with several people who either have physical difficulties or families with relatives experiencing physical problems. When Tim and I were compiling this book, I gained many friends with muscular dystrophy. I had the chance to talk about *ability* with some of those wonderful people whom I befriended through Tim's Facebook page.

Ricky Tsang, a lovely boy with muscular dystrophy from Ajax, Ontario, is the author of a famous book called *RIDICULOUS An Autobrainography.* He agreed to share with us his life experience and we can learn a lot from him.

Costa: Ricky, please can you describe who you are?

Ricky: Thank you, Costa. My name is Ricky Tsang and I'm an author from Canada. I love writing on romance and comedy. I also have Duchenne muscular dystrophy.

Costa: What do you think people with MD have as important gifts to the world?

Ricky: We're nothing special, really. We just have a different set of obstacles, as with everyone else. As human beings, our gift is our capacity to give.

Costa: What do you think they don't have?

Ricky: Everyone has potential.

Costa: What is the secret of your success, as someone with MD?

Ricky: I don't define myself with physical limitations. I'm just me.

Costa: How do you think society treats you?

Ricky: Of course, the ignorant exist, but most people treat me very well.

Costa: Are you satisfied with the facility system to enable people with MD in wheelchairs to access different areas?

Ricky: Yes. There are still some places that don't facilitate wheelchair accessibility, unfortunately.

Costa: Any recommendations for us?

Ricky: You have to fight with everything you have, stand for what's right, say what needs to be said, and die knowing that your life had a purpose. Anything less isn't worthy of who you are.

Yes, "Anything less isn't worthy of who you are," as Ricky told us.

* * *

Alexandre Mejat is a lovely man from France with a PhD in Biology, whom I found through the Muscular Dystrophy Association, as he is actively involved in activities that support those with physical challenges. He was very touched with the idea of writing a book that will help readers to focus on the strengths we have as humans and help us avoid hosting fear within us.

Alexandre willingly shared the following while responding to my questions:

> My name is Alexandre Mejat. I am president and cofounder of Myopathies.info and I am personally affected by muscular dystrophy. Too often, people equate motor disability with mental limitations, whereas most of the time, it is the opposite. I personally know brilliant people with muscular dystrophies who compensated their physical disability with intelligence. In my case, I am a Physician Doctor (PhD) in

> Biology and I worked four years in the USA at the National Institutes of Health before coming back to France to work on muscular dystrophies physiopathology."

Costa: Do you think people with muscular dystrophy get sufficient space in the community to show their skills?

Alexandre: In the work world, most of the time it is hard to obtain the few necessary adaptations to be able to work as anyone else can. We really need to have laws and more positive examples to convince companies and administrations to hire disabled people and give them the tools to be as (and even more) efficient than anyone else !

Costa: Are you satisfied with the respect (value) that is being provided to people with muscular dystrophy?

Alexandre: I have travelled a lot and seen that the situation is very different from one country to another. I really hope people with muscular dystrophies will come together to improve the situation everywhere in the world!

Costa: In a few words, what is a successful story that you have achieved to benefit someone with muscular dystrophy?

Alexandre: I realized that muscular dystrophies are rare diseases and that most of the time people and families directly affected find it difficult to meet other people in a similar situation. I created an online community, called Myopathies.info (http://www.myopathies.info) where neuromuscular patients can share their everyday life experiences in a safe and private space.

Costa: Any recommendation to the world?

Alexandre: As Saint-Exupéry would say: "The essential is not visible to the eyes." Open your heart !

Regarding Fear and Caring

"Caring about others, running the risk
of feeling, and leaving an impact on people,
brings happiness." – Harold Kushner

Fear is a preventable visitor and it acts within us when we allow ourselves to be the host agent. When we are consumed by fear, our strength and ability to change our life positively are obscured. After the death of my father, which impacted all of my family, we could not predict what our life would be like. Without our father, my family was struggling to survive in the midst of the unsupported Rwandan refugee status we were living under, in the Democratic Republic of Congo.

My mom, as a young widow, struggled daily to provide even one meal for us. My mom would repeatedly tell me and my siblings that our sufferings were caused by a lady named Helena who had been [unfairly]accused of having "witched" my father. When my mother had that thought, she couldn't even cook for us or go to the market to run her daily small business. She felt herself to be a useless widow who couldn't provide anything for the five children she had to raise at that time. My mother mistakenly believed that her peace was being held back by Helena.

As we rarely had enough to eat even two times a day, my mom would gather us and say, "We are unlikely to regain our lives due to Hutus who killed our relatives in

1959 and made some of us to flee the country."

Most of us grew up believing that we couldn't do anything to make our lives better. Some of my siblings couldn't even imagine the importance of studying. They dropped out of school and my mom understood their decision because of the anger and the hopeless view of life she was holding, full of blames and confusions. These were the fruits of the fearful mind of our mom. I do believe that we harvest a lot from our parents. If parents are peaceful and manage their stress well, their kids can also grow up peacefully.

If we live with fear in our minds we obviously face its consequences. The opposite of this is all about self-empowerment. We must not allow a fearful situation to weaken our lives, as everybody has the strength and ability to discover within themselves the power over this confusion.

What we represent in our minds is simply what we are and what we have. The secret for a peaceful mind is to host peace within us. In my first book, *The Work that Brings Peace in Me*, I took time to talk about the way we can cultivate peace by letting go of fear. When we do not care for each other, we do not care for ourselves. When we are distressed, we become "care-less," and the fact of the matter is that we develop that "don't care" spirit in our minds and then fearfully project that to the outside.

Caring means understanding the potential value and goodness of human beings, emphasizing common human needs, and seeking caring ways of solving human problems. Not caring about our existence is a reaction to the confusion that emanates from a fearful mind.

* * *

It's very rare to see kids with disabilities in African schools. Their parents and their surroundings will tell them that they can't do anything while being disabled. When we are peaceful, we won't see people with disabilities as guilty, embarrassing, shameful, discomforting, weak, something to fear, or lacking of value in the society. This stereotype that we create in our minds nullifies their existence. Because of our fearful minds, which do not perceive *ableness* in people with disabilities, people with disabilities do not venture out of the safety of their family home, and find themselves excluded from contributing to, or participating in society.

But this is a fearful story we project, and not the truth. Everyone has something powerful to do with his or her own life. Everyone has something valuable to contribute to change this world. It's a matter of noticing and believing.

Being an ostensibly "able person" does not necessarily mean being healthy. Deficiency of ability can't be seen in terms of someone's physical or mental attributes that our society has been fearfully using as a discriminatory tool.

Is a stereotype insulting, rejecting, or neglecting? I consider stereotyping a way of devaluing some groups of people because they lack something, or because they appear to be different from everyone else. If you look around in your community, you can see that people with disabilities have as friends only family members and healthcare professionals—particularly doctors or former caregivers (as the new caregivers will be judged unprofessional if they tend to be too friendly with their patients). The rest of the community members will be disinterested in any involvement with persons with disabilities.

At Heathrow Airport, I met a man from the United

Kingdom with a physical disability. I talked with him and he told me that, "Some disabled people here in the UK live in such a hostile situation that they even avoid going out, or using public facilities like parking bays for persons with disability if they don't look disabled."

From my observations, most of us have the habit of looking with pity on those with physical disabilities, and totally think how sad that they need our "assistance" to live. What then happens when we have such confusing thoughts? We can't give credibility or responsibility to someone whom we think "is there for me to help."

Most of us picture people with disabilities as sick, having a poor quality of life, consumers of our resources, requiring expensive assistive devices or services. Many even think that they should not have better places to live other than in nursing homes; that if they lived in private homes, they would need to be under constant supervision.

When you check into many companies that provide support services to people with a disability, you may find the word "independent" being used in a misleading way.

It is important to notice that when we treat people with a disability as disabled people, as a separate group of society—as people who don't contribute, as weak, or sick, we automatically exclude the ability to be independent. We assume that persons with disability are not capable of thinking for themselves, or of doing many things for themselves.

In many developed countries and even in the most powerful countries with high human rights ratings, people with physical disabilities are still accommodated in long-term care facilities that cause them to live dependently.

* * *

Tim did an advocacy that changed the minds of some authorities and people who watched the video that he made and posted on YouTube. "I want to live in a family home like other young people," he stated in the video. Can you imagine what happens when active-minded, intelligent young people with physical disabilities are hidden away in a long-term care facility, with a hundred insurance benefit restrictions that by their nature create total dependency?

Both people with physical disabilities and those with mental challenges have an equal right to live as independently as possible. Each and every one of us can contribute to this possibility by simply projecting a human sense to others.

During my speaking engagements to caregivers in many assisted-living homes I visited, I carefully worded this question to caregivers: "What are you planning for your clients today?" They responded, "We are planning to take them to the movies, or to a restaurant, etc." and I respectfully reminded them to keep in mind that their clients might like to plan their own activities. A respectful response might start with: "They want to...." I do believe being a caregiver does not mean dictating all decisions for those who live with disabilities.

I have observed many times that companies that provide support for people with disabilities end up planning activities for their "clients," choosing for them what to eat, what to wear, telling them what time to do this or that.

There are a lot of people with a disability who are well equipped with skills and creativity, but they stay in their house. With the new computerized life, people with a disability can perform many tasks that other people do. Despite having muscular dystrophy, my friend Tim does a lot of things on the computer and even more than some so-called "able-bodied people." As someone who likes calculations, I have seen him doing mathematics successfully on the computer and many other things that our entire society values.

"…I have an active mind, and I want to be able to have a career, to be active in the world," Tim stated in his videotaped speech.

Employers often cite the cost of accommodations as a barrier to hiring persons with disabilities. But simply moving furniture can often accommodate employees with disabilities. The vast majority of persons with disabilities who are presently employed require no special workroom accommodations at all.

I had the opportunity to talk with the owner of an art shop. He had a hard time answering my question: "Could you employ someone with disability?" His answer was, "It might depend on the type of disability the applicant has and if my gallery can accommodate a person with that disability."

As with anybody, not working can make you feel isolated, dependent, and rejected from society. The community and motivational aspects of working are often undervalued. Employers can greatly contribute to the quality of life of people living with disabilities by providing them with a wide range of opportunities in which to work. Still, people's minds need to become unconfused and overcome discriminative thoughts in order to see that people with disabilities can work and are capable of performing necessary tasks.

However, there are some companies that should be recognized for promoting independence for people with disabilities, and considering individual abilities by providing accommodations, flexibility, and opportunities. I like visiting the organization Goodwill in Maine that provides opportunities to people with disabilities to perform tasks that are within their capabilities. If Goodwill can do so, then others should be able to provide the opportunity to people with any kind of disability to do what they can.

Most people with disabilities want to work. I have spent time with my friend Tim when he was teaching at a summer camp here in Maine. When I asked Tim why he thought those summer camp organizers accepted his application, his response was that they were aware of his artistic skills, and also they are thoughtful and accepting of people with disabilities. They do not have in their mind the stereotype story that a lot of people have.

* * *

In North America attitudes are changing and community inclusion of people with disabilities is improving, and people with disabilities can sometimes feel much more comfortable in society here. Back home in Africa, people with disabilities are marginalized. Living with a disability in most of the countries in Africa is still purely a hard life experience.

In Africa, people with disabilities, as well as their families, are often excluded by the rest of the community, and receive shameful looks from ignorant critics. The first challenge people with disabilities face comes from culture norms that offer little hope and no real future for them.

Sorrow, horror, isolation and uncertainties characterize the majority of their lives.

One cannot ignore how many African mothers whose kids were born with disabilities are blamed and cursed by their husbands and the extended family for "having brought a disabled into their families." Therefore, to survive with a child who has disability, the mother will prompt that child to begin begging on the street at a young age. In Central and East Africa, except Rwanda where begging is not tolerated, kids with disabilities will be deposited by their mothers at the main entrances of the markets, restaurants, popular streets, or even at churches.

During my 2012 summer trip to Burundi, where I was born, I met a man with disability who was at the main entrance of the Bujumbura Market, and asked him if we could go together for lunch somewhere. He could not immediately accept. He was afraid that there were many people who would question his presence there. I insisted that I wanted just to share lunch with him. He finally accepted, feeling more comfortable after hearing my Rwandan accent. We went into a nearby restaurant. He was crawling, and trying to find a path through a careless crowd of people, and it took us a long time to go a short distance. People were not ashamed to call him *kiwete,* meaning "someone who cannot stand at all." In the restaurant while waiting for our orders to come, I asked him, based on his experience, how people with disabilities are treated in his country.

Shaking his head, he said, "The life of disabled people in Burundi is still horrible. The disabled are not considered as persons in their own right. We are still called *ibimuga,* which means "broken pots." We are treated as scroungers and useless people without any future. Accessibility is not an issue to think about, as it will be boring to my mind, once I take the time to think about it. Public transport is not adapted for us at all and brings a lot of hassle on a daily basis. Disabled people do not have equal admittance to education, healthcare, and information. Their primary rights are not respected at all."

He added that when he was growing up, because of having some physical disabilities that were due to polio that struck his body as a child, opportunities were very limited. A disabled child couldn't go to a conventional school with other kids or access health services. The family would strive to hide him so that the local community wouldn't realize that their family was "cursed." "Today, there is a little bit of changes," he said. "That is why I can go out in public and beg."

* * *

One day I talked with a fellow from India who told me that there was a brother with a disability in his family, who, he remembered, people would stare at because he could not walk by himself. He told me that the brother with the disability ended up quitting school. During the phone call, with a sad voice, my Indian friend told me, "Socially, people with disabilities are not very 'appreciated' in our Indian society. This is not because most Indians are hostile regarding those living with disabilities, but often some are not very thoughtful of disability matters from a humanitarian perspective. Instead of compassion, they often show excessive wickedness, making the people with disabilities feel humiliated. India has today many towers and big buildings, as well as government institutions, that do not give easy access to people living with disabilities because they don't see any reason why people with disabilities would want to visit them."

* * *

My Rwandan cousin's son, Sadiki, suffered from polio at a young age and his legs became weak. At the age of ten he wanted to join us on our way to school, but he could not because he had to crawl, and the road was too muddy during the rainy season and very dusty during the dry season, and that was very cumbersome for his mobility. His father, Deogratias, who is my cousin, is more accepting than most other fathers and families with a child with disability. He loved and supported his son despite the strong stereotyped attitude that he was getting from neighbors and other relatives. "My son did not choose to acquire a disability. That is just the way it is and my heart has received it," he told me.

* * *

When in our minds we fearfully misrepresent people with disability, we become ourselves disabled or weak, and make decisions about integrating them into our society based on incorrect assumptions about their abilities. However, when we become aware that people with a disability have many things they can contribute to the bettering of our world, our minds become strong, and we can believe in the power within us and live positively from the inspiration learned from those with disability.

In North America you can easily see some people with physical disabilities going to the store to shop. They are responsible for selecting and purchasing products on their own. My friend Tim has been a great reference for the best stores or nicest restaurants for many people. I remember one day I was looking for a fresh produce market that I had visited with him and could not remember where it was. After unsuccessfully trying to spot where the market was, I decided to ask Tim. I called him, and he easily directed me and I found the market. When I asked him how come he knows so many places, he told me that his family likes taking him shopping or to different restaurants to eat. "My mother, my dad, uncles, aunts or friends like having a get-together where I participate as well," he said.

* * *

I believe that a peaceful mind is the most creative one. When we are stressed by our fearful mind, we limit ourselves to the access of pathways of peace that God has freely provided to us. **The projector of our life is our mind.** It is very important to carefully verify the quality and sense of what the projector is sending to the outside. This means that the outside has the value of what we project onto it. When we think that our life is controlled by the outside, we become weak and live fearfully. We therefore lose control and can't achieve anything successfully for the reason that we believe someone else has to do something for us so that we can succeed. It's the same thing for our bodies. When we have physical disability there are many things that our minds can easily misinterpret. The interpretation depends on which one of the two conditions our minds hold: Fearful or Peaceful. And then comes the step of noticing.

When our mind is in a **Fearful** condition, we are continuously living in the past by forgetting the power of the present. In this condition, our collective mind is full of fear and tells us many things that discourage our being. It creates dependence by projecting weakness and inability to take action, perhaps because of our physical shortcomings or deficiencies. Our mind can tell us: "Look, you don't have the same physical ability as others, so you can't do anything in your life," and then you believe that. A mind in a fearful condition will tell us we are limited, and we believe that. Sometimes, a fearful mind will use our age: "You are too old (or too young) and you can't do more now." If we believe our mind in a fearful condition, we dump ourselves into a stressful bay. It's very hard to find a mind like Tim's stuck in this fearful condition. So let's talk about the peaceful condition and discover how he manages that.

When you spend some moments with Tim, you can easily double-check with your mind before getting upset at any situation you might be in or personal difficulty you may be experiencing. To one of Tim's caregivers (Connie Johnson, who is also a team supervisor) Tim's experience of life without difficulty is a starting point for everyone to find a self-powered breakthrough.

Numerous caregivers who worked or are still working with people with muscular dystrophy have good memories about the radiance of their clients. Caregivers will tell you how wonderful and inspirational people with muscular dystrophy are. When you are engaged in assisting people with muscular dystrophy, you think about how you would face some changes to your own life. People with muscular dystrophy have a life system that can easily turn your way of living to a "no complaint" way of life. Every day is a new life lesson. It was quite rare for me to leave Tim without learning very important things about life. Muscular dystrophy certainly is not mind dystrophy.

Tim always considers his caregivers as professionals, and he knows that they are there are with him to help in achieving his goals. He feels and notices that, being a caregiver is much more than just a paid job—his caregivers are full of love and compassion. This is what he projects in them and he always notices that it is more than just a job for them.

One day I asked him who he thought could tell us about his experiences of life, apart from his mother and himself. "Doubtlessly," Tim said, "Connie Johnson. Connie knows me well and she is like a second mother."

I have experienced this since I have known Tim. When I wanted to visit him in his apartment in Old Orchard Beach, Connie was the one who gave me directions on the phone. Connie gives orientation to all of his new caregivers. She knows in detail what he likes and what he doesn't like. From Connie you could also become aware of his skills. I remember Connie told me, "Tim does not like to use the same knife used to chop onions for cutting a lemon."

It was a little surprising to Connie to find out that Tim and I are reminding people to see strength and ability in those with muscular dystrophy and in general with any disability, through book writing and introducing people to the pathway of peace.

"Tim is very intelligent and does things carefully," Connie said. I told Connie that we can shape our life by learning from the way people with disability explore their potential to live a successful life.

Many people with muscular dystrophy I met have college degrees, high school diplomas, or are still pursuing their studies. People with muscular dystrophy have an energy that creates a lovely connection with the outside.

Let's together look at the most relevant aspects of Tim's life that can be considered as gifts to ourselves when we manage to live in "The Present."

Humility is not something we can purchase in the store, cultivate in the farm, fish from the sea, or hunt in the bushes. Rather it is a simple discovery within us. We always ignore this and take it as a minor thought. It was amazing to me to notice how all the people with muscular dystrophy I connected with welcomed our relationship. Sometimes it was very difficult for me to understand how their openness was flowing with love.

My friend Tim, whom I never consider to be simply my client, always presents a good picture of humility. He is a friend of small kids, teenagers, young-adults, adults and elderly people. One afternoon when we were walking, I asked him why he thinks everyone who meets him ends up liking him? This was shortly after we had met a lady who ended up hugging Tim joyfully. And after a man came and tapped in a friendly manner on his shoulder and then said that he missed Tim. Sensing my curiosity Tim replied, "I don't know. I think you just be friendly and cool to everybody."

Many of his caregivers have become friends of his. When they get other jobs, they will not leave him completely. Some of them will continue to hold at least one short shift so that they can continue to see and interact with Tim; others will be keeping connected to him through

Facebook, emails, or phone calls.

It happened several times that my kids, who rarely get to spend time with Tim, complained about wanting to visit him. We all know that kids keep in their memory as the reality of the relationship, the first impression they got from meeting with someone. Once you show the kids a warm welcome when you meet them, they will love you forever, and when you do the opposite they will not like you at all.

When I first took my kids, Gentle and Queen, to visit him in his apartment in Ocean Park, Old Orchard Beach, I couldn't predict what was going to happen when they saw someone in a wheelchair, in a position that wasn't common for them to see. However, any fearful thoughts didn't last long due to the lovely and warm welcome Tim gave to them. That changed their minds, and my little daughter Queen, who was two years old, was touching Tim, exploring every room, and petting his cat Zoey.

Gentle, who was seven years old at time, was already on the computer where Tim was teaching him some art designs. Tim was just giving what he has, which is peace and love. He plainly knows that people get from us what we have.

No one can ignore that discrimination is a type of suffering that navigates each minute within people's minds. I do believe that the person who hates is in more pain than the one who is being hated. Here we can take time and meditate on Tim's experience with this issue that has tremendously damaged our society. He doesn't care about race, color, country, sex, age or religion. He welcomes everyone in his life without any discriminative aspect. His caregivers are from different backgrounds and I myself am a real example. When I meet him, I always feel love energy emanating from him during our conversations. He expresses a familiarity that isn't strained. This really gave me a remarkable experience that is the opposite of the fear that is still creating segregation among people from different backgrounds. It is proof that when we are experiencing peace within us, we live in harmony with others.

One day I decided to ask Tim what his reaction might be to something that happened to me and to my son Gentle when we were leaving the McArthur library in Biddeford. Tim looked at me attentively. I told him that I liked borrowing books for Gentle from the library. February 2012 around 5:00 p.m., we went there to get some books. When we were exiting the library, there were six girls standing close to the library's main entrance and all of them appeared to be teenagers. One of them, who looked to be the youngest, spoke loudly to us, "Hi, black dogs." Gentle did not respond the way I did. I asked the girl how old she was and she told me that she was twelve years old. A few days later the same scenario happened to Gentle when he was coming from the school bus stop toward our home. A girl, "Hi, black dog," greeted him. Tim responded to our telling of our experience saying, "hatred is a lack of education and love."

Tim believes that every person has something to give to someone else. You can always notice this when you are walking with him, or during any decision-making discussion. You will hear these words, "What do you think?" When he asks something he will truly wait for your contribution. "What do you think?" Don't deceive him, just give your answer and he will balance. That is in the spirit of valuing everyone's opinion.

Staying Healthy

In Tim's Words

We have a lot of good supermarkets here in the USA, and they are all about the same in terms of grocery items; I can't hide that I like shopping at Hannaford. The simple reason I go there is that Hannaford gives me a lot of choices. It makes me feel comfortable when I am in my wheelchair going around Hannaford's produce shelves, easily accessing the label prices and item details. Hannaford gives me multiple choices and I can go with what I can afford. I also like the arrangement of items and the generosity of the associates who help me tremendously while shopping if I need to know more about items in the store. So when I want to buy something to cook at home, my preference is simply to go to Hannaford.

Good health starts with the decisions you make when you are in a restaurant or supermarket. What you consume is very significant in giving you a good diet. I always like to start my shopping with fresh produce, and it will take time because I like to carefully consider what I am going to get. Though most of the time I don't make a list of items I am going to purchase at Hannaford, when I do, broccoli always comes on the top of my shopping list. Then we'll go with asparagus, cucumber, celery, and spinach. These are my priorities and then will follow fruits. My favorite fruits are mangoes, apples, blueberries, and bananas. I always eat these types of foods to maintain my body in good health.

Oh! I forgot to mention soda water as well. Before leaving Hannaford, I have to make sure I get my 24-bottle pack of soda water. I think you know I drink a lot of water to avoid dryness in my body.

Costa: What about cheese?

Tim (laughing): My mom taught me to avoid a lot of cheese; I like cheese but I am very careful about the quantity and quality of what I consume.

I like cooking at home and rarely go to a restaurant. Some people think I am funny while gathering components for recipes at home.

Costa: Yes, I remember one day you asked me if we could go cook and I was surprised with the recipes. We started by frying skinless all natural chicken, and you requested me to put carrots in it, then broccoli, onion, garlic, tomato and basil. I thought that was all but you said, "Can you put some mushrooms, and some squash and spinach, and a little of bit spice?" I can't remember the other two ingredients we put in it. They were a bit strange to me.

Tim: "Yeah! That was delicious Costa!" (Tim was smiling.)

I learned a lot of recipes from my mother and my grandmother, but also I like checking on the Internet. Then I can print the recipes and can request the caregiver to help me. Most of the time we make good food. That doesn't mean that I have never failed with cooking. The most recent failure, Costa, was when you and I cooked together and we kept discussing different social issues and the fish in the oven was totally overcooked.

Costa: (laughing a lot) Tim that was three months ago, I am surprised that you still remember that.

Tim: Maintaining your body's health means also keeping

track of different contributors of good health. Because of the muscular dystrophy I am living with, I also always live with medication. Every morning I take almost six types of pills, and then in the evening I take two pills. I have to make sure I respect the prescribed medication. I have never minded taking such a bunch of pills every day, as it is part of my life. It doesn't take anything other than commitment.

* * *

Tim knows the secret of how to be in a peaceful condition to manage his life. He doesn't complain at all. He's the type of person who lives much more in "The Present" and enjoys what it brings. He values what he has and uses what we call "limited ability" to do great, unimaginable things. He doesn't think that he has disability. Rather he always thinks of what he can do despite having a disability. That peaceful way of thinking brings a strong willingness to those who have it, and Tim does.

Sitting in his wheelchair, looking straight at the computer, using three fingers of his right hand, he has amazing computer skills. Tim's power of doing isn't stopped by his lack of physical ability, but rather relies on his perfect mind.

His computer has a keyboard directly displayed on the screen. With those three fingers on his right hand, Tim types very fast. He does the same when navigating in different files, browsing the Internet, or designing his art. As someone with English as a fifth language after Swahili, French, Kinyarwanda (my local language), and Lingala, which is a popular language spoken in the two Congos (Democratic and Brazzaville) and other surrounding countries like Angola and Central Africa Republic, it is sometimes difficult to understand 100% of what I am told in English, and some explanations are needed for me to know what is what. There are some products that Tim would like to tell me about, and I can't easily understand what they are. When I ask for an explanation, within a few seconds he will show me pictures on the computer of the products he means. It's another skillful way he can use to accurately communicate. When you are talking about foods, he will quickly find all the health information, and tell you all about it.

"I Am Not Perfect"

In Tim's Words

I am a human; my mind can be fearful and can easily create a loss of control. It happens to me when I get upset, to react negatively, especially when I am not satisfied with what I was expecting. One day I asked my friend Costa if we could find the power cord of my old computer. I had been feeling bad enough to have that computer inactive in my home.

The power cord was misplaced, I am sure accidentally. I don't have the ability to plug and unplug the power cord so that I can keep it in a place where I will find it later easily.

Costa started to hunt for the power cord in my busy shelves. I was going around him with my wheelchair but was still limited to reach some places. My contribution was just verbal. "Costa, can you check in that porch, what about in that closet, please check in that basket, look around that shelf, please check in those boxes," I kept telling him.

Costa did his best but it was in vain. I was really frustrated. Frustration never brings peace, though I could not realize that at the same time. I mistakenly backed up with my wheelchair, hit my laptop and the screen was broken. My frustration doubled and I could not accept what had happened to me.

I was pretty sure if I was not in a wheelchair, I wouldn't have broken my laptop, and maybe it would have only minor damages. It is too hard to make turns in my apartment. That sometimes causes my wheelchair, overloaded with ventilator, tubes, and battery, to hit some stuff while making turns. So I am missing the power cord for my old laptop and broke my current laptop. Costa passionately told me to live in the present and be peaceful.

I came down and went to my desktop and ordered a new cord on Amazon. When the power cord came, it wouldn't fit in the power slot of my old laptop. I was wondering what to do. Surprisingly we found the original power cord in the inside pouch of my old unused backpack. I just learned one of my weaknesses, and how when someone is frustrated they can make mistakes easily.

I know sometimes the computer drives me. I think about how I sit on the computer so much. I'm able to do lots of things with it, but it's not the same as real human contact. I think, "Is it going to help me to be on here, solo, looking at the screen or wall, away from faces and others?"

If I was fully able to physically do what I want, I could get up and move or turn to see others easily. I could interact easily. If I am off the computer I can only drive my chair or recline my seat or elevate my legs. I can't use my CPU or anything else solo, but I am free from the confinement of the CPU, trading one thing for the other.

* * *

Costa's Questions

People with physical challenges know already that everyone has the power to accomplish something despite any challenges they face. They can make changes in their lives. Because they can do so, we need to ask ourselves these questions:

> Should we see a person with muscular dystrophy or with another disability as someone who can't do skillful things? Or as someone who is permanently weak?

There is no mind suffering worse than misrepresenting someone else's weakness in your consciousness. At that time, you become weaker even than the person with a disability.

A teacher from Kelowna in Canada said, "We all have handicaps. Some of us just have a handicap that doesn't show immediately on the outside. For example, a person who has no ear for music would feel very threatened if he were put into a band and given an instrument to play, even if it was only a group of people at a party who wanted to make music together for half an hour. A person with a weak back might look fine at first glance but might also have to excuse himself if a neighbor needed help shoveling some gravel off of his truck and onto his driveway.

When I first meet a person whose handicap is obvious, like someone missing a leg, for example, I feel a little intimidated. I think all of us do. But I immediately focus on the person's eyes, and then I start a conversation about any small matter that seems appropriate at the time. Perhaps some item from the news that day or even just a comment about the weather. I find that the more I talk to a person, any person, the more I think of that person as just a fellow human being.

* * *

Everyone in society has something to contribute, which can positively effect the entire development of this Universe. As I was looking for more contributions to this book, I tried to talk to as many people I could. One day I contacted a young man with muscular dystrophy who willingly committed to participate in the compilation of this book. Michael is an artist living in Maine. His creativity should never be limited only to his home or his body. He has the ability to share, and has something to share. Here is what he shared with us:

> If I had to describe myself I would say I'm a good person, kind of rebellious at times, and I like to push the envelope of everyday life.
>
> I think that if you have muscular dystrophy, if you think about it too much and let it affect how you live, you won't be able to continue. So it's all in your mind. You have to try to think beyond the muscular dystrophy. This disease does not have to define you as a person.
>
> I think people do not realize people in wheelchairs have feelings and want to live a good life just like everyone else. People that have muscular dystrophy look at life a little differently sometimes. I think with a good mind and a good outlook on life, anything is possible.
>
> The secret to my success as someone with muscular dystrophy is to live every day to the fullest. Each day is a new day. Put one foot in front of the other.
>
> Accessibility is one thing many wheelchair

bound individuals face on a daily basis. Access has improved tremendously and most places are wheelchair friendly. Sometimes older buildings are tricky, some of the bars in Portland have steps at the entrances. I try not to let that bother me and just move on. One thing I wish I were able to do, is hang out with my friends more often, but transportation is the issue. Most people can just jump in a car and go and don't even think about it. I sometimes wish I could get my license but it costs a fortune. Even the handicap accessible van I use is double the price of a regular van. Just because it's modified for wheelchair use, why should we be treated differently? I'm sorry it took so long for me to answer these questions; I hope you are doing good and all is well.

It is so peaceful to pause after reading Michael's words. Let's meditate on that and create a sense of personal representation through human equalization.

* * *

One day, I was doing a presentation on self-peace discovery using the theme "look upon your image in someone's face" during a social justice workshop in Wisconsin. There was a professor from a university who was exhibiting some facts on inequality in providing jobs, whereby people with a disability are victimized. He drew up an advocacy project to raise awareness of what is minimizing the value that people with a disability can provide to the nation. I was resistant and asked him to reconsider the core of the problem, which could be found out by asking this question: Which side is suffering more; groups of people who hate or groups of people who are hated? I do believe that, when you hate, you are the one who generates the most hatred and therefore you are the one who suffers. He asked me what he should do. I told him that it would be good to meet those who hate and help them to be peaceful. That is what will end the job discrimination.

Why should we cover up our ability and live dependently? Confidence is what our mind can generate when we trust what we have and who we are. Self-love excludes hatred and expands harmony.

Peace Leads to Creation

Creating something is much easier with a peaceful mind. It is more difficult when we are living with persistent anger, stress or sorrow—emotions I call "Sons of Fear." The deep Peace that Tim has discovered is what leads him to what he is now achieving.

Many people use the word "peace" in different ways. However, the Peace we are talking about here can be a little bit challenging. It's a Peace that for a long time may have been covered over in our minds by Fear. Stress, anger, and hatred are the opposite of real peace. When we don't have space in our minds to help us to question our anger, hatred or stressful thoughts, we end up making a confused decision that we sometimes justify as "the way I can get peace." The result is what I call **Pirate Peace.**

Let discuss little a bit about Pirate Peace.

Without getting into many stories, here is a list of some examples of Pirate Peace thoughts and decisions that can swim in our stressful minds day and night:

1. My parents don't care. For me to live peacefully is to live alone far from them.
2. She/he offended me. For me to live peacefully, she/he needs to apologize!
3. Can't be peaceful, unless I don't have disability!
4. Can't be peaceful, unless I stop being an orphan!
5. Can't be peaceful unless I abuse drugs or smoke cigarettes!

6. Can't be peaceful, unless he or she is killed!
7. Can't be peaceful, while I'm older like this!
8. Can't be peaceful, until I get that clothing, jewelry, house, more money … !
9. Can't be peaceful unless I marry her/him!
10. I feel peaceful only when I talk with people on the same academic level as mine.
11. I feel peaceful when I interact with people with the same social status as myself.

Real Peace versus Pirate Peace

Real Peace is obtained after questioning your mind. It's the result of an interaction between your fearful mind and you. There are many examples that everyone can check with his or her mind and discover whether they are producing Real Peace or a Pirate Peace. Pirate Peace always takes us out of the reality, and rather, creates thoughts that can ruin our lives, while Real Peace always takes us into self-discovery, personal power, and the ability to realize within us the changes needed to turn our lives into lovely ones.

I had the chance to meet a teacher of inquiry who taught me a way you can interact with your mind through a process called *The Work* (see www.thework.com). It is only when we allow our mind to get to the inquiry field that we can spot the blind side built by our fearful mind. The process has four questions and the turnaround. Ask yourself:

1. Is that true?
2. Can you absolutely know that is true?
3. How do you react when you have that thought?
4. Who would you be without that thought?

Then you turn the concept around and find some genuine examples.

I really like and practice the four questions a lot, and most important is the turnaround part. That is where you look at the positive side of the one you think hates you or doesn't care, or even what you think should be done or should happen for you to be peaceful. More to that, the turnaround helps you to look at the other side of yourself and discover the ability in you that can at anytime change your life. It also shows you the power of today that dwells in you. Remember the example of the first stressful thought we mentioned in the list of Pirate Peace:

"My parents don't care. For me to live peacefully is to live far from them."

If we turn this thought around, we would have: My parents ~~don't~~ care. For me to live peacefully is to live ~~alone far from~~ close to them. Genuine examples of this can include but are not limited to: They are still my parents; they raised me; I look like my mom or my dad; my mom tries to call me every week; and other good things they did or are still doing that are being covered by my fearful mind. There comes the Real Peace.

Tim is a good example of the turnaround for his entire life. He always sees himself as strong. He doesn't believe that peace is outside. Rather, he notices day after day that he has the ability to discover that peace which dwells in him, and he does. He sees himself as someone who can easily change everything using his own power and the ability that God gave to him. "I have to use what God gives me," Tim one day told me when I was asking him about an amazing design he did on the computer. Tim has already noticed that everyone has the ability to do something, and he went discovering inside himself for that. When you find Tim on the computer doing some art, if you pay much attention you will discover that he doesn't focus much on the way he is physically, but rather focuses on the "doing" part. That is controlling your situation. Note that we need to be peaceful inside to notice someone's work and bring our minds up-to-date.

Here is a story to help show the difference between Real Peace and Pirate Peace.

Two widows in Africa struggled to find peace regarding the death of their lovely husbands.

The first widow found that for her to remain peaceful the "good decision" was to cut down all the trees that were in the backyard because her husband loved them a lot, and they painfully reminded her of his absence. When she looked at the trees, it reminded her of the death image of her husband. Cutting the trees = Pirate Peace.

The second widow decided to plant a lot of trees and maintained the one planted by her husband because he loved trees. For her, seeing the trees was like seeing the love that her husband had toward her and the environment. Planting the trees = Real Peace.

Real Peace is always there within us and we can access it after noticing that it is possible. I do believe that God gave and gives us peace in its fullness. But we have to remember to cultivate it. We cannot achieve the cultivation of peace until we free our minds from a fearful state of confusion. I find the four questions and the turnaround a helpful way to navigate our minds out of fearful confusions, and get closer to the discovery of Real Peace.

We are able to do, when we want to do

When you are reproving yourself you easily forget to exploit all the power that dwells in you. Your relationship with yourself at this stage doesn't work perfectly. However, there is still a way of hosting peace inside you, by increasing the extent of your focus to the "present." From there comes Power re-creation and rediscovery within you.

There is a Rwandan woman in Africa who can help everyone to double-check with his/her own mind and consequently bring back hope.

Janviere, my wife's lovely cousin-sister, lives in the Eastern region of Rwanda. She has a physical disability that is similar to muscular dystrophy. Her left arm can move only a little bit, but her mind is perfect! She had the chance to finish high school before she acquired physical disabilities. Since I have known her, she is always on her bed. She can't sit in a wheelchair, and the only position she is comfortable in requires her to be on her bed. She sometimes visits her family members who live far from where she lives. The transport is very burdensome. They need to use a vehicle that has room for a bed. Then there is the challenge of being lifted up from the vehicle, into the relatives' house, but this is being done routinely.

She is just an angel. It's hard to know exactly what caused her disability. Maybe due to the less advanced African healthcare system, the origins of Janviere's disability remain unknown.

One summer I had friends visit in Rwanda, from Bonnyville and Edmonton in the province of Alberta, Canada, who support my goal of promoting girls' education in rural areas of Rwanda. They came to visit Rwanda to see activities that they are sponsoring. As the time period they arrived in matched with the time period I was compiling this book, I decided to bring them on the two-hour drive to visit and spend some hours with Janviere, who is always on her bed. When we got to her house, the first thing that was easy to notice was her smile. She was very happy and overjoyed to see visitors coming into her house. "Papa Gentil," she called me. (In Africa, when you have children, it is respectful to call you using your son's name and to avoid using your name.) "I have never had visitors from outside of Africa coming to visit me. This is my blessed day and I am so overjoyed."

Of course as usual, she had to introduce the visitors to her adopted children. It is hard to believe that Janviere adopts genocide survivors' orphans.

More than that, you cannot imagine how Janviere, who is in bed 24/7, can raise those children by her own means.

These orphans who unfortunately lost their parents and relatives, found hope when Janviere, a single mother with a physical disability, opened her heart to them and welcomed them to her home.

I invited Janviere to give you, the readers of this book, her background. Janviere said she was willing to share with you. With a smile and laugh Janviere told me that her disability came when she was twenty-nine years old.

"I didn't know what it was, but it started with malaria that laid me down for two weeks, and then I found my right side paralyzed," she told me. This was before the horrible and fearful 1994 Tutsis' Genocide, when Janviere and her family were among the other innocent Rwandans who were hunted by the militias and government army at that time. "I had some treatment before the Genocide and I could even stand and walk, though with a hand support," she said.

"Unfortunately, everything went wrong. No treatment for three months, the period the Genocide covered, living fearfully, people running, and hiding me..." she said. "...you can imagine the way I was."

"After miraculously surviving [the Genocide] I started to get treatments, but in vain. Nothing changed, and even today I am not sure what kind of sickness it is that strikes me down for years," she said. Janviere found that physical disability "is not at all mind disability." Janviere, who was helped by friends full of love and compassion, decided to bring orphans into her home to share the little support she survives on today. "They are Genocide Survivors like I am. My only wish today is to help these five orphans to build their future," she told me calmly.

I knew that in Africa and particularly in the countries where I lived, in Central and East Africa, there are no food stamps or financial assistance for people with disabilities. I asked Janviere about the overall support for people with physical disabilities. She told me that Rwanda has tremendously raised awareness about the equal values and rights that people with disabilities should have in the society. "Nowadays, we people with disabilities aren't as much excluded in the society, and this is because of the Rwandan government's support to nullify the stereotype in people's minds," she added.

Janviere is such a gift to those who live hopelessly, and dedicates her life to support those who are extremely in need by helping them to build hope and focus on self-resilience.

I was very curious to know the reaction of my

American friends who visited Janviere in the Eastern region of Rwanda. None of them knew who Janviere was and whether or not she had critical medical conditions, but they did know that she was a Genocide Survivor. I approached one of them, who is a psychologist whom Rwandans named *mahoro,* meaning Peace, for creating happiness for many Rwandans by being friendly to them and talking to so many in buses, in the villages, and the markets. I wanted him to tell what his first reaction was when he saw Janviere, and then after interacting with her, any lesson he might have learned from Janviere.

He took a deep breath and said,

> It is unbelievable to have survived Genocide and being hunted while having a disability, as Janviere has. When I saw her lying on her bed, with a peaceful smile on her face, it raised a hundred questions in my mind. Even before we were introduced, I was really touched to see her. Though confined to her bed, she could stretch her left arm high enough to ensure she hugged the visitors with a warm heart. It was challenging to meet Janviere and hear she had survived genocide. However, she created clarity in our mind and we were all at ease. It was so amazing and inspiring to see her, despite her paralysis, raising orphans in her house. The house was warm with mutual interaction and happiness. We saw how she was coordinating everything by whispering in an orphan's ear, welcoming us to the dining table and feeding more than ten people. As we were all enjoying

the meal, I could also see the happiness on her face, from the bed where she was lying. Meeting her was a high lesson that teaches us how much we need to value whatever ability we have. Everyone is able, and if Janviere, who is paralyzed on one side, and lives with horrible memories of the Tutsis' Genocide, can smile, then WHY NOT ME? She is a hero, full of Love and prosperity and I want to see her again as she is a life changing example! Thank you Costa!!"

* * *

What makes us to be so negative in our lives? When this question arose in me, I searched for a pathway to peace. When we live with so many excuses and complaints, we discount the value of our being and place confining limits around ourselves. What follows? Uncontrolled actions, rebellion, complaints, anger.

Everyone is equipped with power. In my past, I repeatedly would see myself as trapped in a miserable life— as someone who was raised in a poor African country by a widow with refugee status, who was barely able to provide one meal a day for all eight of us children. When I was growing up I kept recalling when I was a victim of malnutrition and I had so many excuses for not living positively due to the painful life I had experienced.

However, the day came when I challenged my mind with the question, "Whose business is it when I live with negative thoughts?" When I began to question my mind, then the power within me showed up. I discovered that power and started telling myself a new message in the

Present, "I love me, I feel happy, I have the power to have and achieve my goals."

When we drop stories and excuses in our daily life, we surely create the space to progress and live our lives focusing on the Present. This power can't be purchased in any store, or be transferred from anyone else. However, we can discover it within ourselves and live peacefully.

A friend of mine who was a constant cigarette smoker told me how he could not quit smoking, until the day I asked him, "Whose business when you smoke and whose business will it be when you quit smoking?"

Discovering the power of doing within us is a great change-tool for joy. Excuses and complaints amplify fear within us and degrade our ability to experience joy. Despite being wheelchair-bound due to muscular dystrophy, my friend Tim decided to dethrone fear from his life and gave that place to the Power that dwells within him.

Complaint is a product of FEAR.

A friend of mind asked me one day what I understood to be FEAR and I responded that it is a **F**orce that **E**liminates our **A**ptitude **R**eprehensively. One of the ways to learn how we can live fearlessly is to begin to understand how fear debilitates our ability to shine. When fear knocks on our door, we do have the choice to do a self-inquiry on its appearance. When we don't take the time to question the presence of fear, we end up by accommodating it, and it leads us to a confusing life of complaints and negative ideas. Fear weakens our ability to discover other, more peaceful and positive ways of seeing a situation. When we let go of fear, we are free to see the world at large from a peaceful, loving place, and to acknowledge everyone's ability to contribute to life, and to value every living person. The opposite of FEAR is LOVE. A Fearless life means a Loving life.

* * *

We must not write people off and label them as sick or disabled. We must give everyone a chance to grow and live as full a life as they can. If our fear causes us to strike them down as faceless categories at the first sign of inconvenience, disfigurement, or any kind of "different," we are failing them as well as ourselves.

Just knowing other people's stories of joy and sorrow can kindle understanding and compassion, and hopefully, some form of positive action in our world.

Our hope is that Tim's story awakens us to a larger understanding, and helps us to discover, as Tim has discovered, the power of peacefully Living the Present.

In this way of Living the Present, Fear can be overcome.

www.ingramcontent.com/pod-product-compliance
Lightning Source LLC
Chambersburg PA
CBHW071217200326
41519CB00018B/5565